THE HEART AND
VITAMIN E

THE HEART AND
VITAMIN E

by EVAN V. SHUTE, F.R.C.S. (C), MED. SCI. D.

and the medical staff of
The Shute Institute of Clinical and Laboratory
Medicine, London, Canada

KEATS PUBLISHING, INC.
New Canaan, Connecticut

CONTENTS

INTRODUCTION

No substance known to medicine has such a variety of healing properties as alpha tocopherol (vitamin E). It is unique. That has always been one of its major difficulties: It is too useful for too many things.

One would never expect, in the day of the antibiotics or tranquilizers or cortisone, that the possession of multiple values would be a hindrance to the acceptance of alpha tocopherol, but it is.

Medical men who were originally taught that alpha tocopherol was a "fertility vitamin," controlling the tendency to miscarry noticed in some women, later learned to their surprise that it could resolve scars in claw-like hands, and often refused to believe it was more useful still for diseases of the heart and blood vessels. That was too much.

All important medical discoveries have sounded improbable or even a bit fantastic to both doctors and laymen alike. Think back on some of the older discoveries and how odd they must have seemed at first. Fancy taking a mold from the air, growing it on artificial media, then injecting a solution containing it into muscle to treat an overwhelming bacterial infection in the abdomen, lungs or tonsils! It sounded so fantastic that it took fourteen years and the Second World War for medical men to *give it a trial!* However, we have all conveniently forgotten our first misgivings in our current enthusiasm for penicillin.

1

Insulin is but one of a host of similar examples. Imagine extracting a fluid from the pancreas of a slaughtered animal and injecting it under the skin of humans to help the body use any sugar not properly handled by the patient's own pancreas. That is what Sir Frederick Banting did and then announced the fluid to the medical world as insulin.

Alpha tocopherol (vitamin E) was at first received with the same unbelief and for the same reasons. Once understood, however, it will be as universally used as are the antibiotics (penicillin or streptomycin, tetracycline) and insulin.

Vitamin E is useful for a variety of diseases which at first seem totally unrelated. But there is one factor that they have in common—a local decrease in oxygen supply because of injury to veins, arteries or capillaries, or because of internal organ derangements. Understand this, and the reasons become obvious for the use of tocopherol in such apparently dissimilar conditions as nephritis, coronary thrombosis, burns and diabetes mellitus.

Skepticism is no new thing. The difficulties encountered by penicillin we have already cited. One would have thought its virtues were obvious from the first, and readily demonstrable. BCG vaccine, after clinical trials made upon millions of people over the last fifty years, still has an uncertain future. The use of anticoagulants in coronary heart disease, even after a carefully controlled study carried out by hundreds of the leading medical men of 16 university hospitals on 1031 patients has been followed by scores more.[1]

One can go back further into medical history

and recall the story of X ray. When X rays were discovered morality brigades were formed at once, designed to resist such a destruction of decency and privacy. A London firm made a small fortune selling X-ray-proof underwear. An attempt was made in New York to legislate against the use of X rays in opera glasses in theatres. All this is now forgotten, but it illustrates that some of the best medical advances have had tardy recognition.

Such medical and public caution is wise, particularly in a day like ours when medical advances are so numerous and, like the Salk vaccine for polio, often take long to adjudicate. But once the evidence accumulates to the height that studies on alpha tocopherol have reached, and when the diseases it can alleviate and prevent are so menacing and general, the debate should not be prolonged further. For in the meantime thousands upon thousands suffer or die needlessly while easy help lies within their reach.

Hence this little book. We want to be sure that the medical profession, as well as the patients dependent on it, know what help is available. We have spent many years in bringing our findings before doctors. We have published a profusely illustrated textbook on the subject for scientists and medical men in general. We have lectured on our findings before the British, Canadian and Ontario Medical Associations and the National Medical Association of the United States, as well as before many international medical meetings. This is the customary procedure with new medical observations, and this custom we have observed. Now here are the facts in everyday language.

Chapter 1

WHAT IS VITAMIN E?

Vitamins have always been labeled according to the letters of the alphabet. This was a good device as long as it was a simple matter of A,B,C and D. Now since there are M,P, and even lower letters in the series, and, what is worse, several D vitamins and even more B vitamins, this system of nomenclature has aroused much criticism. Whenever possible, scientists now differentiate the components of the vitamin B complex by speaking of thiamine chloride or riboflavin or pantothenic acid or niacin. They even prefer to speak of ascorbic acid in place of vitamin C, although only one type of C is known.

Vitamin E is also a complex of several factors: the alpha, beta, gamma, delta, epsilon, eta and zeta tocopherols. For all practical purposes gamma and delta, perhaps epsilon, can be ignored at the moment. Alpha, beta and zeta appear to be the factors of most use to us in medicine, and alpha overshadows the

rest. Hence in this book we equate vitamin E to alpha tocopherol, since "vitamin E" is merely a kind of
medical shorthand or slang for the alpha substance.

What is a vitamin? It is a food factor, present in
minute amounts in certain foods we eat, and essential
for proper nutrition. Each one of the many so far discovered acts in a way characteristic for it and for no
other. It may act on one set of tissues only, perhaps
on one small focus in the body. Some, it is true, have
certain resemblances to one another in their effects,
for example, alpha tocopherol and pyridoxine (a
fraction of vitamin B). Some are helpful to one another or, as we say, "synergistic." An example of
good companions are vitamin A and alpha tocopherol.
Some are antagonistic, such as alpha tocopherol and
natural vitamin D (because of the unsaturated fats in
fish liver oils, the commonest source of D).

For a long time vitamins were supposed to be
harmless in any amount. Now it is known that over-
doses of such factors as nicotinic acid (part of the B
fraction) or vitamin D can be given to certain sus-
ceptible persons, and that a high dosage of ascorbic
acid (vitamin C) may be poorly tolerated by some
stomachs. High doses of the tocopherols may develop
the same problem, or produce diarrhea or a skin
rash. Some people have trouble taking thiamine.

Presumably most vitamins take part in the activity of the enzyme systems of the body. Recent work,
for example, suggests that alpha tocopherol is involved in the activities of such a substance, called cy-
tochrome C. In the heart it is involved in enzyme
systems of a complex nature called nucleotidases and
oxidases. As yet these biochemical processes are far

from adequately explored. Suffice it to say that vitamins appear to be potent in small quantities, are essential to the enzyme systems of the body, and are often involved in an integral way in the metabolism of foods.

Vitamin E (alpha tocopherol) is known to act as an anti-oxidant, hindering the undue or too-rapid oxidation of fats. It hinders the production of tissue peroxides, hence the deposition in tissue of pigment "clinkers" (incompletely burned or oxidized food factors). It is also a factor in the utilization of both carbohydrates and proteins, the other main constituents of all food.

In recent years the concept has evolved of the use of vitamins as drugs, without regard to their activities in minute quantities in food. Thus *huge* doses of vitamin D, far beyond those ordinarily demanded by the body, have been used by physicians treating arthritis. Huge doses of vitamin C have been used in an anti-infective role. Huge doses of niacin have been used as a dilator of blood vessels. Huge doses of thiamine chloride and of B-1 have been used for neuritis. This involves the so-called "pharmacodynamic" action of these substances—in short their use as drugs, not as replacement only. It is in this sense that we usually administer vitamin E nowadays, especially for cardiovascular conditions, using doses far larger than the so-called "minimum daily requirement." This has opened up a whole new field in vitamin therapy, which is no longer regarded as being of value purely for the relief of major deficiencies or for replacement. We are now in the epoch of *"megavitamins"* (as christened by Professor Linus Pauling).

Since the exact chemical structure of many vitamins is now known, some have been made syntheti-
cally to set beside those isolated from natural
sources. Most of our early clinical work was done
with synthetic alpha tocopherol, for example. We
learned from this experience that it was the alpha
fraction of vitamin E that was most significant thera-
peutically. Probably synthetic ascorbic acid is now
more widely used than natural vitamin C. Certainly
synthetic vitamin K is used almost exclusively, since
new K-like substances have been found to be more
potent than the natural vitamin K originally discovered. Not only that, but knowledge of the structure
formulae of vitamins has enabled researchers to
predict that substances with somewhat similar molec-
ular configurations might duplicate some or all of the
roles that certain vitamins play. Hence the inter-
esting studies indicating how far selenium, methy-
lene blue or diphenyl-p-phenylenediamine can
replace alpha tocopherol, for instance.

Vitamins can act much like hormones, alpha tocopherol resembling progesterone in its effect on
pregnancy, for example. Or they can be antagonistic,
just as a female sex hormone and vitamin E have
very different effects upon the vaginal wall or blood
clots in the legs. Unravelling the chemical nature of
these agents has gone far to indicate the parts they
play, occasionally has enabled man to improve them,
and certainly has suggested more and more roles in
which they may prove valuable.

A BRIEF HISTORY OF

ALPHA TOCOPHEROL OR

VITAMIN E

In 1933 when we began our studies on the effects of vitamin E, we used an ether-extracted wheat germ oil. In those days it was difficult to protect it from the rancidity which destroyed its alpha tocopherol potency; this problem continued when we used a fresh, cold-pressed wheat germ oil prepared in linseed oil presses and correspondingly unpleasant to taste. The oil had to be dated and kept cold to make sure it was strictly fresh and therefore potent.

In 1939, the "synthetic" product came on the market. It was quite stable and very concentrated. Naturally, it at once became the League of Nations standard. Its major difficulty was that in large doses, it was sometimes poorly tolerated by the stomach.

About a year later, natural tocopherols in concentrated form in gelatin capsules came on the market. These were prepared from cheap cottonseed oil or soya bean oil, were then methylated to produce the

active alpha form of tocopherol, and on a price basis
alone were soon able to dominate the commercial
field. They still do, particularly since they are more
potent than the synthetic form, weight for weight,
and in large dosage are more agreeable to many
stomachs.

We doubt that wheat germ oil is sold today as a
source of alpha tocopherol, since a modern vitamin E
capsule containing 100 international units contains
about 240 times as much alpha tocopherol as a typical 3 minim capsule of wheat germ oil. If any one
does buy the wheat germ oil for its tocopherol content, it is probably useless. Vitamin E is both curative and protective. But it is silly to feel that these
properties are to be found in doses of the substance
so small that they would scarcely protect a grasshop-
per from coronary thrombosis. There is no excuse for
unnecessary disappointment with tocopherol therapy,
and perhaps for needless deaths among the unin-
formed.

This brings us to other problems concerning
sources of alpha tocopherol in the market today in
the host of preparations called "vitamin E," "vitamin
E concentrate," or a multitude of trade names.

In Canada, a Federal regulation passed in April,
1948, compelled standard labeling of preparations of
alpha tocopherol in terms of the League of Nations
International Unit. However, Dr. David Turner, of the
Sick Children's Hospital in Toronto, purchased bottles
of alpha tocopherol capsules at random from open
shelves in Toronto drugstores. To his great surprise,
the labels bore no close resemblance to the alpha
tocopherol content. Indeed, the labels might claim

SOME PREPARATIONS OF VITAMIN E ON THE MARKET*

Label Claim	Material Used	Actual Potency (Int. Units)
100 mg d, alpha tocopherol	100 mg #1 with 588.2 mg Type IV (natural) −17%	92
100 mg d, alpha tocopherol by biological equivalent	68 mg #2 from 272 mg Type VI (natural) −25%	92
100 mg dl, alpha tocopherol	100 mg #3 synthetic	68
100 mg dl, alpha tocopherol by biological equivalent	73.5 mg #1 from 432.4 mg Type IV (natural) −17%	68
100 mg dl, alpha tocopherol by biological equivalent	50 mg #2 from 200 mg Type VI (natural) −25%	68
100 mg dl, alpha tocopherol acetate− Int. Unit	100 mg #4 synthetic	100
100 mg dl, alpha tocopherol acetate− Int. Units−by biological equivalent	108.7 mg #1 from 639.4 mg Type IV (natural) −17%	100
100 mg dl, alpha tocopherol acetate− Int. Units−by biological equivalent	74 mg #2 from 296 mg Type VI (natural) −25%	100
100 mg d, alpha tocopherol acetate	100 mg #2 from 400 mg Type VI (natural) −25%	136
100 mg mixed tocopherols	294 mg Type IV (natural) −34% M.T.	46

*Dr. David Turner, Sick Children's Hospital, Toronto
Published in Toronto Newspapers, April, 1969.

values seven to ten times higher than were warranted. The "best" products were one quarter of the strength claimed. His findings are listed in the table below.[2] Dr. Turner was the N.A.S.A. consultant who found that the spacemen in the Gemini study lost much of their red cell mass and at least five-sixths of their plasma tocopherol in four days' time. This was ascribed to the high oxygen level of their other-worldly environment. Dr. Turner suggested that vitamin E be added to their diet.

That has also been true in Europe, as far as we can find out. Over there the synthetic vitamin E has had things pretty well its own way on the Continent, and the natural, made by highly reliable firms, has held sway in Great Britain and Italy. Both have been thoroughly reliable preparations, properly assayed and accurately labeled.

In the United States, in the face of severe competition in an increasing market, there are hundreds and hundreds of brands, selling for a wide variety of prices and differing label claims. Some well-meaning physicians have been disappointed in the results from some preparations they have prescribed.

We ask you to make certain of the product you buy. There *are* reliable brands on the market; we have no facilities to test every brand, nor do we intend ever to set up such a thing. But the worthy manufacturers are known, and the unworthy product soon makes itself obvious. As of now no prescription is needed at Canadian drug stores and only in some states in the United States. Of course, reliable brands are available at health food stores.

Chapter 3

ALPHA TOCOPHEROL

IN OUR FOOD

One is often asked the question: "What foods should I eat in order to get enough vitamin E?" This is difficult to answer helpfully, for many foods contain vitamin E that do not contain much alpha tocopherol. It is alpha tocopherol that matters in cardiovascular disease, pregnancy, diabetes and such conditions.

Vitamin E is a constituent of cereal germs. Therefore it is found principally in oils extracted from such germs, such as vegetable margarines made from soybean oil, wheat germ oil, corn oil or cottonseed oil. These oils, of course, readily turn rancid, and the least trace of rancidity promptly destroys their vitamin E content. At the beginning of the twentieth century, millers found that a stable, exportable wheat flour could be produced if the germ were separated from the rest of the kernel. In that moment an intercontinental grain trade was established and a corresponding deterioration of public health began, for alpha tocopherol could be obtained from no other common food source in comparable amounts.

Look about the table in an average North American household. One finds gamma tocopherol in the greens of salad, a little alpha tocopherol in the whole wheat bread, more alpha tocopherol in any good *vegetable* margarine being used—and that is about all. Is it any wonder that years of accumulated alpha tocopherol starvation produce lesions in the hearts of nearly all animals so deprived? Consequently, vitamin concentrates have become the order of the day. And because one is catching up on years of alpha tocopherol starvation, studies indicate that now one must overstoke the furnace in order to secure the results that should have been achieved by many years of low heat.

It is characteristic of alpha tocopherol feeding that large amounts must be eaten in order to induce small rises in blood levels. For example, to double the blood content one must increase the intake 40 times. Once a human being takes 100 mg of alpha tocopherol daily one must increase that intake by 500 percent in order to raise the blood level by only 9 percent. The assimilation of tocopherols in healthy persons is less than 50 percent, and in the unhealthy may be much less. The bowel excretes about 75 percent of the dietary intake of alpha tocopherol. The urine excretes almost none (less than 1 percent).[3]

It is difficult to say what is the "normal" requirement of alpha tocopherol in food. It has been estimated that typical American diets contain 10 to 25 mg of alpha tocopherol per day. Studies done in

Rochester, New York, by Harris and Quaife suggest that the alpha tocopherol intake of pregnant women averages about 6 to 13 mg daily.[4] The United States National Research Council recommends diets averaging about 6 mg of alpha tocopherol daily. Now subtract from this the alpha tocopherol lost in cooking, as in deep-frying which can destroy 70 to 90 percent, or in baking pies which destroys 25 to 75 percent, and one sees that the alpha tocopherol content of "normal" American diets can be very close to zero.[5] Hickman has estimated it generously at "not more than 10 mg daily."[6]

Chlorine dioxide has now replaced agene as the most commonly used flour improver in the United States. This commercial chlorine dioxide treatment of flour reduces the tocopherol content by about 70 percent. The tocopherol in this bleached flour is destroyed in baking bread.

In order that readers can see at a glance what foods are rich in alpha tocopherol and what foods are not, here are tables derived from Quaife et al below.

Apples with skin contain the most tocopherol of all fruits, which are poor sources at best. Commercial canning and storage cause large losses of alpha tocopherol.

Vegetables are also very poor sources; sweet potatoes and turnip greens top the list. The tocopherols of such vegetables as turnip greens, carrots, and celery are almost 100 percent in alpha form. On the other hand the tocopherol of legumes such as navy beans and peas contain almost no alpha. However vegetable oils extracted from celery, sweet potatoes or tomatoes may contain much more alpha toco-

TABLE ONE

TOCOPHEROL CONTENT OF FRUITS AND VEGETABLES*

Tocopherol Content

	mg/100 gm fresh material alpha	Percent of total tocopherols alpha
Fruits:		
Apples	0.72	more than 97
Bananas	0.37	more than 93
Grapefruit	0.25	more than 96
Oranges	0.23	more than 96
Vegetables:		
Beans, dried navy	0.10	3
Cabbage	0.06	55
Carrots	0.45	100
Celery	0.46	more than 96
Lettuce, head 1	0.29	67
Lettuce, head 2	0.29	54
Onions	0.21	81
Peas, green	0.10	5
Potatoes, sweet	4.00	100
Tomatoes	0.27	75
Turnip greens	2.24	more than 97

*Quaife et al—*J. Nutrition* 40: 367, 1950

pherol than wheat germ oil. Ordinary table potatoes are a poor source of vitamin E, but kale and parsley are among the richest sources of total tocopherols.

In most cereals only half the total tocopherols are alpha, except in oats, where they are almost all alpha. Polishing rice removes 75 percent or more of its vitamin E. Whole wheat flour loses about half its total tocopherols when milled to white flour. The man who eats 8 slices of white bread per day would thus get 0.5 mg of total tocopherols as opposed to 2.6 mg from whole wheat bread. The older bleaching processes, moreover, destroyed as much as 70 percent of the half or third of the total tocopherols remaining after milling.

TABLE TWO

TOCOPHEROL CONTENT OF SOME CEREALS

	Tocopherol Content	
	mg/100 gm fresh material *alpha*	*Percent of total tocopherols* *alpha*
Cereals:		
Cornmeal, yellow	0.84	49
Oatmeal	1.94	92
Rice, brown	1.20	50
Rice, polished, converted	0.35	61

The next table, indicating the alpha tocopherols in meat, fish, poultry and dairy products, shows how poor most of them are in this respect, except for eggs. Two eggs supply 2.4 mg of tocopherols, about

60 percent being alpha tocopherol. Haddock, salmon
and sardines are good sources. Cow's milk is poor.
Processing it to make cheese, butter or evaporated
milk does not alter this. But milk from pastured
cows may have four times as much tocopherol content as stall-fed cattle.

Everyone should pause to ask himself this question: "If I cannot get enough alpha tocopherol in my
food, and if this semi-starvation goes on for forty to

TABLE THREE
TOCOPHEROL CONTENT OF
MEATS, FISH, POULTRY AND EGGS

	Tocopherol Content	
	mg/100 gm fresh material alpha	*Percent of total tocopherols alpha*
Meats:		
Bacon	0.44	more than 83
Beef, steak	0.47	more than 75
Beef, liver	1.40	100
Lamb, chops	0.62	more than 81
Pork, chops	0.63	more than 89
Fish:		
Haddock	0.35	more than 90
Poultry:		
Chicken	0.21	more than 84
Eggs, whole	1.16	58

sixty years, and if the heart of nearly every animal that has yet been tested undergoes degeneration when that animal remains deficient in this vitamin for much shorter periods of time than that, what *must* have happened to my heart over the course of the years?" Perhaps the cure for that heart could be a hair of the dog that bit it. Why not try vitamin E (alpha tocopherol)?

Animal fats are uniformly poor sources of vitamin E, unlike vegetable fats and oils. Of the latter, cottonseed, peanut, rice, bran and wheat germ oils have 70 to 85 percent of their total vitamin E as alpha. Soybean oil has only 10 percent alpha. Chocolate, peanuts, beechnuts and palm oil are also rich in alpha tocopherol.

The maximum daily alpha tocopherol obtainable by the average American at his abundant table is about 19 mg—the more likely actual level being 14 mg.

Thus the average American daily food intake can be assessed for its alpha tocopherol content as follows:

Commodity	Average Consumption	Intake of Alpha Tocopherol
	gm/day	mg/day
Fats and oils, including butter	80.8	7.87
Grain products	212.5	1.78
Meat, poultry and fish	196.4	0.99
Potatoes and sweet potatoes	142.9	0.84
Eggs	58.4	0.68
Dairy products, excluding butter	535.6	0.58
Green leafy and yellow vegetables	141.7	0.50
Dried peas, beans and nuts	19.9	0.43
Citrus fruits and tomatoes	130.5	0.35
Other fruits and vegetables	290.8	0.12
Coffee, tea and cocoa	23.6	0.06
Sugar and syrups	131.7	0.00
Totals	1,964.8	14.20

Since alpha tocopherol constitutes 90 percent of the total tocopherols in the human body, the latter seems to pick it up preferentially. This agrees with all the workers who have found alpha tocopherol to be *the* significant tocopherol in human treatment.

In man and animals the intake of polyunsaturated fatty acids (PUFA) and the duration of relative tocopherol starvation, determine the requirement of alpha tocopherol. Thus Horwitt, in his initial studies at Mt. Elgin, gave a man 3 mg of tocopherol per day for five years, then found 60 mg per day over many months barely returned him to normal blood levels.[7] The human requirement can thus vary six-fold. About 5 to 7 percent of the population (as high as 30 percent in Uganda) are estimated to be vitamin E-deficient. Deficiency may take years to show up, whether in calves or humans. Humans, for example, develop brown bowel (the bowel is brown on opening the abdomen and rectum. This is due to pigment deposition.) but only after two years of vitamin E deficiency.

The American National Research Council's recommended dietary allowances now state that adult requirements vary from 10 to 30 mg per day. Herting believes that therapeutic preparations should contain 45 to 75 I.U. and notes that various workers have used up to 600 mg daily for malabsorption syndromes.[8]

Be it noted that daily doses ranged around 3 and 10 I.U. or mg until our studies appeared.[9] Now doses of 1,600 to 2,000 I.U. daily are not rare.[10]

Chapter 4

WARNING AGAINST
SELF-MEDICATION

Patients themselves have most to suffer from self-administered alpha tocopherol. No one can say: "Because you have blue eyes and weigh 140 pounds you should take 200 mg per day." Medical treatment was never that easy, and it is not now. The dose for any given patient or disease condition varies, and must be altered with regard to the patient's initial blood pressure, rheumatic or thyroid or diabetic history, and the progress of his condition. Patients who have been treated by us realize this. We have long warned our medical confreres, too, that vitamin E, like any potent drug, can be dangerous. That is the measure of its potency, indeed. Too much insulin or digitalis or arsenic or "sulpha" can kill. That does not mean one should not use insulin or digitalis. It does mean that such a preparation must be used cautiously and properly, by someone familiar with its difficulties as well as with its advantages.

More and more physicians are learning about alpha tocopherol and the technique of its administration. We publish a medical journal, the *Summary*, yearly, which is filled with articles on this subject, written both by ourselves and by physicians from Paris to Florence to Leamington Spa. This is distributed to all physicians who ask for it—and about 22,000 copies are now sent out annually.

However, it is not easy to find among family doctors one who is sympathetic to the use of vitamin E. What to do?

You could be your own detective. Ask around. This is not nearly as difficult as it was ten years ago. The developing orthomolecular consciousness is obvious and almost unimpeded. Vitamin E-sympathetic doctors are there. Look for them.

There have been exhibits of photographs of our results at such international medical meetings as the Third International Symposium on vitamin E held in September, 1955, in Venice, Italy, and similar exhibits have been on display at annual meetings of the British Medical Association, the Canadian Medical Association, the Ontario Medical Association, the American Osteopathic Association, and others.

In 1954 we wrote a larger book for physicians, with the collaboration of authorities from Ireland, Italy, France, the United States and our own country, Canada. It was illustrated in color. This was called *Alpha Tocopherol (Vitamin E) in Cardiovascular Disease*. It has long been out of print, after several reprintings. It was the first book on the subject, also the first book on cardiovascular disease written in Canada.

The first edition of this book you are reading was published in 1956. It has sold about 191,000 copies. It has replaced the larger and more expensive text, now out of print.

Chapter 5

HOW VITAMIN E WORKS

As we have said, no substance known to medicine has such a variety of healing properties as alpha tocopherol:

1. It reduces oxygen requirement in tissues. Therefore, where diminished blood supply or diminished available oxygen is the principal or secondary cause of distress, vitamin E (alpha tocopherol) must be of real help.

2. It melts fresh clots by fibrinolysis. This is best seen in cases of *acute* phlebitis where the clot may occasionally disappear in as little as five days. A "thrombus" is a clot in a vein or artery—"thrombus" means that a clot or thrombosis has formed. It can be a state rather than a tiny clot.

3. It rather rapidly increases the extent of collateral circulation. Where an area is deprived of blood supply, it helps the smaller blood vessels in the

area to open up and so return blood supply along alternative channels to the limbs or area cheated of circulation.

4. It dilates capillaries (the smallest size of blood vessels), which bring the blood to burned areas, for example. This delivers more oxygen to the region where it is most needed.

5. It occasionally removes excessive scar tissue. No other medical agent does this.

6. It prevents the overproduction of scar tissue and, more important still, prevents scar contraction as wounds heals. By contraction, large scars produce deformities which often necessitate skin grafts. Deformities often can be prevented by using vitamin E, and the need for skin grafting disappears.

7. It mobilizes and increases platelets, which are vitally involved in the normal blood clotting processes.

8. It decreases the insulin requirement in approximately one-quarter of "adequately" treated diabetics who have blood vessel complications in the limbs.

9. It is one of the regulators of fat and protein metabolism.

There is also evidence to indicate its value in preserving the soundness of capillary walls, in stimulating the growth of skin over wounds, the excretion of urine, the power and activity of muscle, and in preserving the walls of the red cells in the blood. It also has many veterinary uses (see chapter 37).

In General:

Where clots (thrombosis) or deficient circulation due to artery or vein disease constitute the main or an important part of a disease it is specifically indicated.

Specifically:

Its property of oxygen conservation enables alpha tocopherol (vitamin E) to be of use in gangrene, coronary and cerebral thrombosis (clots), diabetes mellitus, congenital heart disease, arteriosclerosis, Raynaud's syndrome (characterized by spasm of vessels of the fingers), phlebitis, intermittent claudication, systremma, and other leg problems due to poor circulation, athletics, mountain climbing, aviation, abruptio placentae, threatened miscarriage.

Its fibrinolytic powers (melting clot) prove useful in thrombosis, after childbirth, after operations, during and after coronary infarctions.

By dilating capillaries, it helps all patients with impaired circulation, such conditions as arteriosclerosis or thrombosis.

By its capacity to strengthen capillary walls it can help nephritis (Bright's disease), acute rheumatic fever, purpura, retinitis (a degeneration of the back of the eye), threatened abortion, and premature detachment of the afterbirth.

In resolving scar it helps Dupuytren's contracture, chronic rheumatic fever, strictures, Peyronie's disease.

By increasing platelets it earns a role in thrombocytopaenic purpura, thrombosis.

By acting directly on diabetes it is especially useful in such dreaded complications as gangrene.

Its effect on skin repair renders it useful for burns and other wounds, chronic ulcers, skin grafts, many types of skin disease.

In stimulating urine excretion it occasionally aids acute and chronic nephritis, heart failure, dependent edemas generally.

As a stimulant of muscle power it helps athletes, congenital heart disease, heart failure (especially on the basis of chronic rheumatic heart disease).

As a preservative of red cell walls it has been advocated as a routine for blood banks in hospitals, extracorporeal circulation machines, etc.

Its effect upon the metabolism of fats and proteins is profound and fundamental in all bodily processes, digestion and nutrition especially.

Nowadays many millions of women take a contraceptive pill daily. This can lead to many unpleasant consequences, notably phlebitis, and prophylactic measures should be taken. Vitamin E is that precaution and every woman on the contraceptive "pill" should be taking vitamin E every day if for no other reason.

Chapter 6

EVIDENCE OF HEART DISEASE

The heart is a pump whose work it is to force the blood through the arteries everywhere in the body and to receive the return flow of blood at the same rate. If either side of the pump fails in its work, symptoms of that failure appear. Conversely, the ability of the heart to carry out its pumping action efficiently under conditions of stress and work is the best measure of its well-being.

An obviously damaged heart may nevertheless function normally for years. This is the usual story in chronic rheumatic heart disease. On the other hand, an apparently well heart may suddenly break down under sudden stress and damage—as in the case of a sudden shutting-off of blood supply in a coronary artery by a clot.

Symptoms of heart disease, then, are symptoms of failure in the pumping station. If one can walk at a normal rate both on the level and up a moderate incline, and for a considerable distance, then the heart is obviously a pretty efficient pump. Therefore, the distance one is able to walk quickly before symptoms appear is often a fairly accurate measure of the heart's efficiency. The commonest symptoms of poor heart action are discomfort, or pain, or oppression in the chest on exertion, or shortness of breath, or swollen legs or fluid in the abdomen or chest or a combination of these.

Several other factors influence the rate of onset of these symptoms, for example: overweight, anaemia, a recent heavy meal, and, of course, the condition of the muscles. These all contribute to possible trouble.

Pain in the chest (angina pectoris) when caused by a poor heart, has this characteristic, then: That it is brought on by exertion or excitement and relieved by rest; or by nitrogylcerine. Short, shooting or stabbing pain is therefore usually not ascribable to the heart, nor is the usual heart "ache."

Of course, collections of fluid in the chest, with a cough, shortness of breath on slight exertion, or the need to sleep propped up on pillows, are evidences of serious damage and failure to function of the left or expelling side of the pump. On the other hand, a swollen, tender liver or swollen ankles or pulsating neck veins may be evidence of failure in the right or receiving side of the pump. Both of these types of incompetence we call "failure" or, more accurately, "congestive failure."

These symptoms, particularly the mode and time of onset and their relationship to exertion, may constitute the most important evidences of heart disease.

The electrocardiogram may be a very useful aid to diagnosis—in fact may be the only means of making it in a few cases, as, for example, in certain types of blockage of conduction of the nerve impulse down through the core of the heart. However, *the electrocardiogram may be, and often is, perfectly normal in spite of the presence of very definite or even advanced heart disease.* In coronary disease or if coronary thrombosis is suspected a repeat electrocardiogram is taken after a week or two months.

The X ray is very helpful in determining how much injury a rheumatic or hypertensive heart has experienced; however, it often does not indicate in any way the existence of past disease, or the amount of improvement which may develop subsequently. In our clinic the X ray is usually repeated in twelve to eighteen months in the case of enlarged hearts, for it tells us if any enlargement found is of long standing, and if the right side or left side, or both sides are mainly involved.

Too much exposure to X ray is potentially dangerous, one must remember, and many doctors are careless about this whether examining teeth or chests.

Chapter 7

CORONARY HEART DISEASE

The report: "He's had a coronary," conveys word to everyone of a sudden heart accident, often immediately fatal, sometimes permanently crippling if the patient survives. If he lives, he exists only to wait in apprehension for another attack. Everyone knows that, like strokes, these tend to repeat. It should therefore be immediately stated that there are two major types of coronary disease, occlusive and sclerotic (thick walls and clots), and that the drastic occlusive kind described above is a novel and distinctive product of the twentieth century. It is this kind that is probably preventable, but if it has occurred, it should be treated *at once* with vitamin E, in addition to standard therapy. Nothing else offers comparable hope of minimizing damage that has already occurred.

There are two coronary arteries which tap the oxygenated blood from the aorta, our largest artery, immediately after it leaves the heart. They run over the surface of the heart, sending branches into the muscle and thus supplying the heart with the oxygen it must have to carry on its work. Unfortunately, in two vital areas of the body, the heart and the brain, the branches of such main arteries do not interlock or join with each other as richly and freely as they do everywhere else. Sudden or gradual obstruction of a coronary artery or cerebral artery in consequence can be very serious. Some of the heart muscle is completely deprived of blood by such an arterial stoppage as has been mentioned and that segment of muscle must therefore die. Around each such area is a layer of cells which just escapes death, called the "zone of injury," and around this area again are cells which are less seriously injured but are temporarily impaired by the sudden deprivation of blood oxygen. This last area is therefore called the zone of hypoxia (lack of oxygen).

Look at the list of activities of vitamin E that were listed earlier and it will be obvious that here is one situation where *all* the enumerated uses of this agent have specific application.

Alpha tocopherol dissolves the clot or thrombosis partially or completely—if the clot is fresh. Thus it may even prevent death of part of the area otherwise doomed. It decreases the oxygen need of the whole zone of injury and preserves much of its normal structure and function. It returns the zone of hypoxia toward normal and helps the whole injured heart to work more efficiently. Proof of this is in the more rapid and more complete recovery of heart power in patients adequately treated from its earliest stages with vitamin E, and more specifically, by the rapid return to normal of many grossly abnormal electrocardiograms in such patients. Recurrent attacks tend to be prevented by continuous use of alpha tocopherol in *full dosage*—only enough is enough.

Unfortunately, immediate treatment with alpha tocopherol is denied to many patients as yet. This is one of the cruellest results of the slow medical acceptance of vitamin E treatment for heart disease. When a coronary patient survives the initial attack, even if he displays a good deal of heart impairment, he is still an excellent subject for vitamin E treat-·ment. Of course, the infarct (the area killed by lack of oxygen) can never be restored to normal. However, the zones of injury and anoxia are the areas of heart muscle that cause many of the symptoms, and these are still theoretically amenable to treatment and salvage.

One of the characteristics of vitamin E therapy in all forms of heart disease is the latent period between the beginning of treatment and the full development of the patient's specific response. There is no demonstrable help short of a week or ten days; full benefits are obvious in perhaps one month, and continue thereafter. Deaths from the initial shock in those with massive clots or thrombosis in those hearts ill prepared for such an onslaught are scarcely affected by the use of alpha tocopherol. But the good effects noted above are obtained in almost all persons who survive the initial week.

One other point must be stressed here. Normally the danger of a clot forming on the inner wall at the site of damage and so lying relatively loose in a chamber of the heart is great. With vitamin E this danger is diminished and usually absent. Embolism, as the detachment of such a clot is called, is very rare in our experience.

This paragraph should be of utmost interest to every male and to most females. Coronary thrombosis kills nearly half the men who die over the age of forty-five. Only two cases of clotting in the coronary artery were described prior to 1900 in spite of the great interest in and careful examination of coronary arteries at autopsy for decades before that time. It was not found again until 1912! Clearly this is a disease of the twentieth century with no direct relationship to coronary arteriosclerosis (hardening of the arteries), an old and well-recognized disease. There is considerable evidence to support this novel view. The coincidence in time between the beginning and rapid increase of this disease and the beginning of and steady progress of alpha tocopherol deprivation in our diet is too obvious to need stress here.

However, there is a second type of coronary disease, also very common, which is due to the progressive narrowing of the coronary arteries, usually with advancing age. This type has been studied and described for many years and because it causes the same symptoms, although they tend to be lesser in degree and more gradual in onset, is sometimes confused by both physician and patient with the clotted or obstructed type previously described in this chapter. There is no direct relationship, although of course the patient with this type of gradual coronary artery arteriosclerotic damage can also develop thrombosis. Occasional superimposition of a clot upon the sclerosis led many early observers to suppose that this gradual narrowing of the arteries predisposed the sufferer to an inevitable thrombus or clot. The best evidence that this is not so is that this type of arteriosclerotic coronary artery disease seems to have been *decreasing* during the last four decades while coronary clotting has been on the sharp increase.

In either case, the symptoms that develop are those of oxygen lack. With increased demand by the heart for oxygen during exertion or excitement or anger, the arteries just cannot carry enough blood to transport it—thus a state of hypoxia (lack of oxygen) develops. The hypoxic heart causes pain, usually in the chest, often extending to the left shoulder and down the left arm. This is called angina pectoris. It may or may not be preceded or accompanied by shortness of breath (dyspnoea). The patient is scared into immobility, the heart quietens down so that it needs less oxygen, the blood supply catches up to its needs *at rest,*—and the pain disappears.

Alpha tocopherol works ideally here, chiefly by oxygen conservation. However, its clot-preventing and clot-dissolving characteristics are really of more interest to the patient.

Provided that blood pressure is normal and there is no old rheumatic damage to the heart, a good 60 percent respond well to an adequate dose of a properly labelled product—taken faithfully every day as long as the patient wishes to remain alive and well.

Chapter 8

ANGINA PECTORIS

Angina means choking or strangling, and angina usually implies pain in the chest as well. By common
consent this term has come to be restricted to pain
due to heart disease, usually caused by constriction
of the coronary vessels in spasm or due to sclerosis
(hardening). It was first described in the 18th century by Heberden, as everyone knows. Other chest
pain is called dolor pectoris.

Even fifty years ago angina was comparatively
rare. Now it is extremely common.

The history alone usually makes the diagnosis. It
is a pain produced on effort and ceasing with rest. It
can be of any grade of severity and, although usually
located in the region of the heart, can be felt far from
that area. It is commonly confused with neuritis in
the chest wall, a condition aggravated by breathing
or movement or coughing, not necessarily associated

with bodily exertion, and characterized by tender areas between the ribs, in the chest wall itself.

Attacks of angina may continue for many years and may finally lead up to a coronary attack of more serious nature, either thrombosis or the sclerotic obliteration of the vessel's bore that is technically called "occlusion." The pain may be crippling in its intensity and frequency, and prevent a patient from working or even walking.

The usual treatment is by nitrogylcerine or its derivatives. The patient is urged at the same time to do less. He already knows he must, because exertion brings on the savage pain. Unfortunately nitroglycerine gives relief only briefly, and must be taken frequently on that account. It gives mere alleviation of symptoms. It does nothing to heal the underlying disease.

Vitamin E (alpha tocopherol) seems to be the best treatment to date. It often fails—but more often it succeeds. And it succeeds by attacking the underlying physical problem. It dilates blood vessels whose closure is a factor in causing the anginal distress. It enables the heart muscle, staggering under its load while living on a reduced blood supply, to utilize the oxygen of that blood more effectively. It is somewhat comparable to putting the patient in an oxygen tent. Even patients who do not get complete relief often get enough help from alpha tocopherol to do more than before, perhaps enough to get along on and to maintain an interest in life.

Even where pain is unrelieved it is still important for anginal patients to take alpha tocopherol. These patients tend to develop a coronary clot or thrombosis. This food factor is the best insurance against such clotting, and the *safest* that can be provided.

Since many such patients have some elevation of blood pressure, the cautions about dosage that we repeatedly urge must be borne in mind.

Chapter 9

HYPERTENSIVE HEART DISEASE

In Chapter 15 you will find a discussion on high blood pressure and its relationship to heart disease. The heading in this chapter is a general term covering a variety of conditions in which obvious heart disease and an elevated blood pressure are intimately associated.

Recurring attacks of acute nephritis, or an acute nephritis which gradually becomes chronic, is often associated with an elevation of blood pressure which may persist after clinical evidence of the kidney disease has almost or entirely disappeared. Since hardening of the arteries in the kidney usually follows a protracted high blood pressure, it is impossible in advanced cases to tell which occurred first. Hypertensive heart disease is often found in women giving a history of toxic pregnancies, (*see* chapter 34) or recurrent pyelitis, or in male patients in later life, who have chronic prostatic obstruction with "back pressure" on the kidney.

Occasionally a spasmodic type of very high blood pressure develops in patients with a peculiar and rare type of tumor occurring just above the kidney, in the adrenal gland (pheochromocytoma). Removal of this tumor is followed by a return of the blood pressure to normal.

Therefore treatment of hypertensive heart disease involves a thorough search for the cause of the hypertension. Obviously any causative or associated chronic pyelitis, or prostatic obstruction, or disease of such sort must be corrected if possible.

We found early that alpha tocopherol in daily massive doses led to rapid improvement in a good share of the cases, with disappearance of the symptoms of failing heart action and even with a reduction of some blood pressures toward normal. In many cases, of course, improvement in the heart was associated with a maintenance of the same unfortunate blood pressure level. However, in an important number of cases, approximately one-third, the pressure actually rose *initially* on such dosage, often to dangerous heights. Continued experience has not helped us to find distinguishing features in these hypertensive heart cases which would allow us to foretell which patients would respond safely and in which cases the pressure would rise on such levels of medication. Hence we have been compelled to treat all cases slowly and gradually, unless under careful daily surveillance in the hospital. Unfortunately this means that instead of clinical improvement in the heart in three or four weeks, at least three months and often much more must elapse before any improvement at all can be expected.

We have evolved a safe dosage schedule, which causes no harm, allows us to help the fortunate third in three months, the less-fortunate third whose pressure neither falls or rises in a little longer time, and the remaining third to an important but not as complete degree over a still longer period. Obviously some hypertensive heart patients cannot be helped by alpha tocopherol therapy—and we have more "failures" in this group than any other. However alpha tocopherol is still indicated in all such cases. It is still good treatment. It is still the best insurance such patients can take against the blood clotting they all fear—the clots which are called "strokes" or apopolexy. This alone justifies its use.

Remember, like all potent drugs, in proper hands it is safe and often highly effective. These are patients who need every help medicine can provide. They should not overlook one of the most valuable—alpha tocopherol.

Lately we have used the diuretics extensively in hypertensive patients, with improved results in many examples of all the categories discussed above.

Covered with a hypotensive agent thus, one can fairly safely risk the initial high dosage of alpha tocopherol that such patients really need.

We can now use higher doses of alpha tocopherol in hypertensive patients if necessary and control effectively any elevation of blood pressure with the new antihypertensive drugs. In mild hypertension modern diuretics suffice. In moderately severe cases Inderal, Hydralazine, Ismolin, Declinax, Catapres or others are added. And in very severe and malignant hypertension very potent drugs, such as Diazoxide, Arfonad, sodium Nitroprusside are used in a hospital setting.

Rauwolfia preparations are used often but they should be used with care or avoided in women. Some recent reports have suggested that these drugs may make women more prone to develop breast cancer. If this is confirmed this will change their role.

Chapter 10

CONGENITAL HEART DISEASE

More and more children are being born with defects of development. Indeed the number of such cardiac defectives has almost doubled in the last thirty-five years. Such defects are usually multiple, and may cause death in the first hour or month of life. Many of these patients, however, live for some years. Some even survive into middle age with hearts that have been defective since birth. Skilful surgery can remedy many more such conditions than was once possible and return the patient to normal health. For example, many "holes" in the partitions between the chambers may be repaired successfully. However, a great many cases of congenital heart disease are not amenable to surgical correction.

An occasional patient with congenital heart disease shows very little disability. But the majority have serious symptoms, greatly diminishing their ability to live normal lives as well as their life expectancy.

Symptoms are those due to oxygen starvation of all the tissues and hence a decrease in the ability of every tissue and organ to function normally. Exertion of any kind increases oxygen need, and then the symptoms of oxygen lack are increased. In a large proportion of cases, blood returning to the heart, which has given up its oxygen to the tissues and which should be sent through the capillaries of the lungs to re-load oxygen, instead is shunted to the left side of the heart. The patient is thus shortchanged. This cheated, bluish blood is mixed in the left chambers of the heart with the bright red, luckier blood which has gone through the lungs. Both are then pumped to the muscles, organs and tissues of the body. When one-third or more of the body's blood is "unsaturated," or deprived of its quota of oxygen, the skin and mucous membranes turn noticeably blue. This is called cyanosis.

Therefore, the symptoms of congenital heart disease are chiefly those of shortness of breath on exertion, poor growth, susceptibility to infections, particularly of the nose, throat and bronchi, an inceased susceptibility to rheumatic fever and sub-acute bacterial endocarditis, to clots in the vessels of the brain, lungs and extremities—all of this with or without blueing of the skin and mucous membranes. In some cases the child finds he breathes best in a squatting position and assumes this after exertion. Heart failure (dropsy) is a frequent complication. Antibiotics for complicating infections, and digitalis for this "failure" have been the main medical agents available for such patients until alpha tocopherol began to be used.

Alpha tocopherol brings a unique value to these cases. It cannot, of course, do anything to improve the structural defect. However, it can reduce the need of the tissues for oxygen just as in animals tested at high altitudes. It can reduce or remove cyanosis, aid growth, and prevent clots from forming. For those cases which are operable it is a vitally important pre-operative preparation which seems to prevent shock at operation and helps convalescence.

Alpha tocopherol also may be needed to supplement the partial help surgery gives the type of heart defect called "the Tetralogy of Fallot," in which four types of heart defects are found together at birth and the little patient is seriously circumscribed in all his activities. It seems to be safe in any dosage in such cases. It usually must be given throughout life, of course. It opens up a whole new avenue of hope to these pitiful patients.

Chapter 11

ACUTE RHEUMATIC FEVER

There is an obvious parallel here between this dread disease of children and the grave damage to the heart which so often follows it, and acute nephritis (Bright's disease). Both follow an acute streptococcal infection of the throat in about ten to fourteen days. In rheumatic fever the tissues involved are the serous membranes covering the brain, the linings of joints, and the lining (including the valves) of the heart. When the lesions are numerous in the coverings of the brain the patient may develop "Saint Vitus's dance." When the linings of joints are chiefly affected one has "rheumatic fever," "inflammatory rheumatism" or "growing pains." Girls are affected more than boys, red heads more often than blondes, and blondes more often than brunettes. In any case, the important lesions develop slowly and often at first silently in the valves of the heart, and the patient may experience months or years of apparently

47

normal health before the heart insidiously begins to fail. When it does, this is due to two factors: the direct damage to heart muscle which often accompanies the disease, but varies tremendously in different patients, and the strain upon the heart muscle due to the effort needed to pump blood through a narrowed or leaky valve or valves.

Unfortunately nearly half the sufferers from acute rheumatic fever have no knowledge of their illness because their brain membranes and joint linings are not so inflamed as to give symptoms. In such patients the first indication may be the detection of a murmur many years later at an insurance examination, or beginning failure of the heart to function normally on exertion. Such a person may be an excellent athlete in his or her teens, but a cardiac wreck at thirty-five. The chronic stage is gradual and prolonged, and many such patients live as chronic invalids for years.

Fortunately this disease is decreasing in frequency owing to the use of antibiotics and the sulfa drugs in treating sore throats with fever. Treat the sore throat adequately and rheumatic fever is unlikely to develop. Once rheumatic fever has occurred the antibiotics are nearly if not quite useless in the acute phase.

Treatment up until 1946, largely by salicylates, has been almost helpless to prevent heart damage—it has merely helped to make the patient more comfortable while languishing in bed for months and making a slow, fatigued and often illusory clinical recovery.

Without going into the details of the basic lesions in rheumatic heart disease, it is probably sufficient to say that they lend themselves ideally to alpha tocopherol therapy provided that, as in the case of phlebitis and nephritis, treatment is begun within a day or two of the onset of symptoms. In such cases all signs and symptoms may disappear within a week or so. Each day that elapses decreases the speed and the completeness of recovery and may prevent it. The alpha tocopherol dosage used must be large and the product reliable, of course.

Several research groups have reported on the effects of ACTH or cortisone treatment in acute rheumatic fever. However, these agents have not proven any more effective than salicylates (aspirin-like drugs) and are frequently accompanied by dangerous and unpleasant side effects. Also the so-called "rebound phenomenon" frequently follows their discontinuance. All the old symptoms recur, and this may leave the patient even worse than he was in the beginning, certainly more discouraged. We do not use them, except in severe cases.

The real effect of an acute attack cannot be assayed until several months or years have elapsed. Alpha tocopherol should be taken continuously in appropriate dosage, for this disease is often a progressive process.

Chapter 12

VITAMIN E IN
CHRONIC RHEUMATIC
HEART DISEASE

The patient with chronic rheumatic heart disease is
all too common, and is a distressing sight. He begins
by being mildly short of breath, puffs too readily on
mild exe.ti..., .urns a little blue, develops swollen
ankles. Later, as he slides steadily downhill, he finds
he can do less and less, is more breathless, has more
swelling, is more discolored, and is told he is "in failure." He becomes able to do less work or none, may
even be confined to his home or to bed, and reveals
to his physician waterlogged lungs, an enlarged liver,
a large heart and swollen legs.

His physician gives him digitalis in the early
stages of his disease, to slow down and strengthen
the heart beat. Later on he may give diuretics to increase urinary output and decrease swelling. But he
is fighting a losing battle unless alpha tocopherol is
also used. It should always be a part of the treatment
of such patients.

50

It *must* be taken under medical supervision, however, for this powerful agent can do harm as well as good if unwisely used, as is true of any other potent agent used for this condition. We strongly urge people not to treat themselves if so afflicted. They would not take digitalis or diuretics on their own. Why should they feel that alpha tocopherol is an exception to the rule about self-treatment?

We always urge that dosage begin at a very low level, and be increased only slowly and under repeated careful observation. The dosage may never reach a level at all comparable to that used in other cardiac patients. When these warnings are ignored, patients can be thrown into deeper failure.

The proper dose, found for each patient by careful medical study, must be maintained indefinitely; otherwise the patient returns to his original unsatisfactory status and steady downhill progress. This point should also be emphasized: alpha tocopherol is "treatment" for these patients, not "cure" in the sense that a fracture heals and is thereafter "cured." It resembles insulin, for example, which must be taken for the duration of life. Perhaps that is because tocopherol is a food, and food remains a continuing necessity for all of us. Moreover, most of these adult rheumatic hearts are and have long been permanently damaged, are badly scarred, have thickened linings, and heavier, thicker muscle. Nothing could possibly restore them to "normal."

But alpha tocopherol, by its oxygen-conserving powers and its effect in directly stimulating muscle and other such activities, enables what remains of that poor heart to function best—not normally, perhaps, but at the best that is possible. It is a unique help, but it does not restore that scarred and irreparably damaged heart to its original status.

It is merely the best single treatment for hearts of this type.

It may often need to be taken together with digitalis or diuretics. But usually, as it is kept up, less of the digitalis is needed, sometimes none. Indeed, one must watch people taking vitamin E for signs of too much digitalis ("digitalis intoxication") on doses of the latter they have long tolerated well. Fortunately, physicians generally are aware of this.

In brief, then, chronic rheumatic heart disease is a prime indication for taking alpha tocopherol (under close medical supervision), indefinitely, and with or without the classical drugs so long used for such heart disease.

Chapter 13

THE CUSTOMARY TREATMENT

OF HEART FAILURE

Those classical medicines it is the custom every-where to use for heart illnesses are used by us in exactly the same manner and for the same indications as by others, with the simple addition of vitamin E. For example:

(1) *Digitalis*—Many patients taking alpha tocopherol need less digitalis than before; some need none. The indications for the use of digitalis have been established for 180 years. It is *not* a useful drug for a large fraction of all heart patients, however.

(2) *Nitroglycerine*—gr. 1/100 or 1/200 may be used for intense pain, one or two being placed under the tongue and repeated in five minutes if necessary. It is not habit-forming.

(3) *Diuretics*—should be used in heart failure patients if the weight increases two to six pounds above their lowest weight (which must be ascertained).

(4) *Aminophyllin* suppositories by rectum are often helpful, alone or combined with diuretics. This drug has no effect on the vessels of the heart but does help the asthma often associated with heart disease.

Salt restriction is necessary only if the swelling of the ankles, liver or lungs is helped by this measure, in which case one may replace it on the table with granulated kelp or a salt substitute.

Water should be temporarily diminished in patients with swelling but need not be restricted with patients taking a low sodium diet. Except for short periods, water restriction is usually not valuable and may be dangerous as well.

Avoid iron, excessive fats and perhaps estrogens. The only medicine that should not be used with vitamin E is inorganic or metallic iron. Iron is not harmful in itself, but it seems to prevent alpha tocopherol from being absorbed. The iron in food (spinach or raisins, for example), probably is not harmful. Animal fats such as lard, cod liver oil or butter should be used only sparingly, as they increase the body's requirements of alpha tocopherol. Estrogens are tocopherol antagonists, particularly in problems in the breast, vagina and with phlebitis. *"The pill"* if fundamentally just another estrogen. *It should be "covered" with alpha tocopherol* as we have insisted for years.

Do not stop taking alpha tocopherol. The most frequent mistake is to assume that when a patient gets worse or does not improve or requires treatment for another condition (such as a cold), he should interrupt tocopherol treatment. This is almost never the case. Vitamin E can be taken with any medicine except iron.

Signs of overdosage are rising blood pressure, palpitation of the heart and increased fatigue. The cardinal sign of underdosage is failure to improve in the expected time. Complete absence of definite improvement is unusual except in the worst cases. Even then, with attention to detail, the most surprising results are frequently seen.

Indigestion is a symptom occasionally encountered by people taking tocopherols. For this we advise skimmed milk, "casec," or a change of type of the vitamin. If one cannot take the oily gel he can try the succinate or acetate form and vice versa. Alpha tocopherol is best taken in the middle of meals, but may be taken at any time. If taken in one dose at bedtime, one knows he has had his dose for the day and need not wonder if he has taken all of it or not. He dodges the iron in breakfast cereals by this separation. There are brands which are not satisfactory, and we restrict ourselves to the use of those which we know to be of reliable potency. May we repeat: Be sure of your brand.

Frequently people lose their sense of improvement in two weeks after stopping alpha tocopherol, just as a diabetic regains all his old troubles as soon as he stops insulin. People may feel well for several months after stopping tocopherol therapy—and then have a repetition of coronary thrombosis, for example. This might not have occurred had such people continued to take the average maintenance dose necessary for continued health.

It is a real problem that patients given tocopherol often feel so well and vigorous. They act as if they were sixteen years old again. Remember to mix vitamin E with commonsense. If it could make you sixteen again, we would all be sixteen.

Occasionally, but more rarely nowadays, doctors complain: "There are so many opinions about vitamin E." We would suggest that you talk to other doctors who have used an adequate dose of a reliable preparation of alpha tocopherol. Many opinions that one hears expressed are not based on actual experience with this treatment. Improper dosage or a product of low potency in this or any other agent used in treatment would render any trial misleading.

Recovery from angina can be hastened by dilating the arteries and lowering the pressure inside the chambers of the heart by nitroglycerine sucked under the tongue or the inhalation of an ampul of amyl nitrite both of which act quickly and briefly. Isordil, cardilate, or coronex in doses of 5 mg sucked under the tongue act similarly to nitroglycerine and are better tolerated by some patients. The relief from angina pain may last longer with these drugs than with nitroglycerine. For more prolonged action a dose of 10 mg of these drugs is being used. The tablets are swallowed three to four times daily. Peritrate also belongs to this group. Persantin is sometimes used as a coronary artery dilator but it is less efficient in bringing a rapid relief in angina. Inderal (propranolol) is being extensively used in angina. It acts by blocking excessive nervous stimulation to the heart, so that the heart is not exposed to a sudden urge to faster action in response to extra exertion or to emotional stress. It should be given under medical supervision and it is contraindicated in patients with bronchial asthma or with an existing or pending congestive heart failure and in heart block. Many cannot tolerate it.

Just as a diabetic takes insulin forever, so a heart patient must take alpha tocopherol as long as he lives. The physician does his very best to advise the lowest dose which he feels is consistent with safety. This is an individual matter in each case. Remember that alpha tocopherol substitutes for a chronic dietary deficiency, as well as being useful in its own right as a pharmaceutical agent.

Alpha tocopherol is present in our diet in its natural form in cereal germs, vegetable oils and margarine. By milling cereals as we do and dissipating much of the value of our food by prolonged and excessive cooking, we have taken out of our diet this extremely important element and must therefore supplement it to regain lost ground. The diet we recommend, therefore, is derived from whole grain cereals, especially wheat (freshly ground for cereal and for whole wheat bread), brown rice, beans, soya beans, fruit and vegetables, with a reduced amount of pork and other "saturated" animal fats. Even a large amount of vegetable fats may necessitate more vitamin E intake.

Chapter 14

SURGICAL TREATMENT
OF HEART DISEASE

We are living in a space age world where our whole lives are influenced by speed, rapid transportation and communications and advanced technology. If you so desire, you can eat breakfast in Los Angeles, lunch in New York, have dinner in London and spend the evening at the Moulin Rouge in Paris. Man has split the atom, landed on the moon and sent spaceships to other planets.

Medical science has kept pace too. This last quarter of a century has seen rapid development in modern medical technology. Sophisticated investigative and diagnostic ancillary tests have enabled us to define and correct diseases more readily and easily. Words like cardiac pacemaker, heart catheterization, coronary angiography and bypass surgery have become part of household terminology.

Dr. Boyde Goodyear, of the Shute Institute, investigated the subject of heart surgery in current practice as reported in this chapter.

These recent advances in surgical technique and anaesthesia combined with the development of a method of oxygenating the blood outside the body, the so-called heart-lung machine, have meant that more and more patients with heart disease are being treated surgically. What was previously a desperate venture, used only as a last resort in seriously ill patients, has now become commonplace. Indeed, nowadays some patients who have no symptoms at all are now being operated upon in the hope of *preventing* trouble at a later time. This concept of preventive surgery is extremely controversial.

In acquired heart disease, as distinct from congenital, surgical treatment has become increasingly prominent in the management of conditions such as chronic rheumatic valve disease, coronary artery sclerosis, and cases of heart block related to the insertion of pacemakers.

We believe that surgical treatment should be reserved for patients with disabling symptoms who have not responded to adequate and length medical therapy. Certainly, vitamin E gets us away from many of the dangers and difficulties of surgery and always deserves a trial first. One can always operate. Patients only rarely should be hustled into anticoagulants or surgical measures.

In a rheumatic patient with a scarred, narrowed and leaky valve, surgical treatment usually entails removal of that valve and the insertion of an artificial one. The new valve may become dislodged, or infected, or cause destruction of the blood, or predispose to the formation and mobilization of serious blood clots. The patient is then kept indefinitely on blood-thinning agents by most cardiologists (drugs we deplore and shun), themselves risky. Thus, though dramatic and quick relief of symptoms may be provided, it is not a procedure to be undertaken lightly.

Coronary angiography and cine-arteriograms enable us not only to determine coronary artery stenosis, but the exact degree of stenosis as well. This can be used to determine the need for coronary bypass surgery, a procedure that has become very popular in recent years. The technique has largely replaced previous operative procedures such as coronary endarterectomy, the implantation of a systemic artery to the myocardium, anastomosis of the internal mammary artery to a coronary artery, wrapping the omentum around the heart, sympathectomy, carbon dioxide endarterectomy and the bypass of the ileum to decrease cholesterol absorption. The results of selective coronary bypass surgery have certainly been more encouraging, although it is not without risk.

The technique itself is relatively simple. After the stenotic artery has been identified, a blood vessel from another part of the body, usually a vein from the leg or thigh, is used to form a bypass around the diseased coronary vessel. The blood then flows through the bypass bringing more blood and therefore more oxygen to the heart muscle.

Problems can and do occur. The new blood vessel may collapse or become clogged itself. The graft may be rejected and not function. A heart attack may occur during or after the surgery and could be fatal.

Less controversial is the treatment of chronic complete heart block by the insertion of an artificial "pacemaker." In this condition, because of a fault in the electrical conducting system of the heart, the heart beats very slowly, sometimes only twenty or thirty times per minute. The patient is liable to sudden episodes of loss of consciousness, any of which can be fatal. Drugs are of little value in the long-term treatment of this problem. The heart must be electrically stimulated to beat at a normal rate.

Surgical treatment of heart block with electrical pacemakers has progressed with astonishing rapidity during the last twenty-five years. Callaghan and Bigelow developed a transvenous pacemaker in 1951 that was used to stimulate the patient's heart. In 1959, Furman and Schwedal described permanent pacing of the heart with a catheter placed in the inner lining of the heart tissue.[11]

This procedure has been modified and is now widely used. It is a relatively safe procedure to stitch electrodes to the heart wall, powered by a small pack which can be inserted under the skin of the chest. Recently nuclear-powered packs have been devised which may not require the battery changes normally needed every two years or so.

The operation is done under local anesthetic. An electrode catheter is advanced through a vein (i.e. the jugular vein) into the right ventricle of the heart. Then, under fluoroscopy (X ray), the electrode is placed into the wall of the heart. The pulse generator is then introduced beneath the skin just below the collarbone. This creates the bulge that can be seen in patients so treated. Complications are few, but do occur. Infection, unit failure, thromboembolism (blood clot), and arrythmias (irregular heart beats) can happen.

Although cardiac surgery can be valuable in terms of turning disabled people back to normal lives, much thought is needed before it is embarked upon, perhaps more than is applied at present. Perhaps instead we should be taking steps to prevent atherosclerosis of coronary and systemic blood vessels. A number of causative factors have been identified such as hypertension, diabetes, tobacco, obesity, stress, a high cholesterol diet and a positive family history.

We have become the victims of highly refined carbohydrate foods, frozen TV dinners, fast food chains and junk foods in general. More and more chemicals are added to everything we eat, the long-term effects of which are not yet known. Surely this adulteration of our food is not beneficial, and natural organic foods should be sought out.

An attempt to reduce coronary artery disease by reducing these contributing factors has received much attention over the last few years, but in spite of antihypertensive drugs, insulin and hypoglycemic agents, tranquilizers and low cholesterol diets, the incidence of heart disease has not been reduced. In fact, heart disease is the number one cause of death among Americans.

Chapter 15

HIGH BLOOD PRESSURE

Elevated blood pressure places an added load of work upon the heart and in turn upon the blood vessels. The normal heart can withstand such added work for a relatively long time, since the heart has a great reserve of strength. Similarly, the arteries can withstand an added load while their structure remains normal. However, the reserve of the heart muscle and the elasticity of the blood vessels decrease with age. The added strain borne by the normal heart is borne less well by the aging heart and the aging blood vessels. Of course, any damage to the heart due to rheumatic fever also lessens its reserve and hastens the appearance of undesirable symptoms.

The heart eventually becomes secondarily involved in most cases of high blood pressure and the degenerative change in the arteries is accelerated in most cases because of the added strain of the continued elevated pressure.

At first the heart responds by hypertrophy—a process similar to the development of body muscle in the weight-lifter and wrestler. Each muscle fibre increases in size. The wall of the left ventricle becomes increased in thickness and so is still able to force the blood into the aorta. Such hypertrophy can be seen readily under the fluoroscope in most cases. Later when the burden becomes too great the muscle "fails" and the left ventricle becomes dilated as well as hypertrophied.

It is logical to expect vitamin E to help such a heart and in the majority of cases it does, by supporting the heart muscle directly. Why then does it not always do so?

In the normal cardiovascular system the pressure is maintained at a constant normal level by five factors: the volume of the blood; its viscosity or thickness; the power of the heart beat; the elasticity of the vessel walls; and the peripheral resistance. Of these factors the one chiefly involved and therefore chiefly abnormal when things go wrong is the peripheral resistance, the other factors remaining relatively constant. If the effect of vitamin E were only upon the peripheral resistance, then the effect of treatment would be favorable whenever it was able to lower the resistance to the flow of blood by relaxing the terminal vessels which are in spasm. Vitamin E has been shown to have this effect in animal experiments.

However, vitamin E also improves the tone of heart muscle specifically and this improved tone tends to raise the blood pressure. Fortunately, the spasm in the smaller arteries frequently is decreased by small doses of vitamin E—doses too small to invigorate the heart muscle materially. If this effect is sufficiently marked, the pressure falls and the patient may tolerate a larger dose of alpha tocopherol up to the point where the heart muscle per se is strengthened. The end result and thus the final dosage depends upon the balance achieved between these two conflicting factors. If the relaxation of the arteries is rapid, of good degree and maintained, and the increased action of the heart muscle is in proper proportion, then the ideal situation can be reached—a full dose of tocopherol for the heart with maintained relaxation of the vessels. If, however, the heart muscle tone is increased greatly with relatively little relaxation of arteries, the pressure will not fall enough and may actually rise, in which case a full protective dose of vitamin E may never or only eventually be possible.

Fortunately, in a fair number of patients, with care and patience—great patience on the part of both physician and patient—a desirable balance and result can be achieved, a worthwhile reduction in blood pressure as well as worthwhile support to the heart muscle. This emphasizes the point that self-medication has its dangers and demonstrates why everyone must use alpha tocopherol only under the direction of a physician acquainted with the reservations involved in its use.

Nowadays diuretics and other preparations are widely used for high blood pressure. They are excellent, and work even better in association with alpha tocopherol.

As a preventive measure against the apoplexy that so often develops with high blood pressure, alpha tocopherol plays a particular role. Every hypertensive should be given it, if for that reason alone.

Chapter 16

GENERAL FACTORS INFLUENCING

THE ACTION OF ALPHA TOCOPHEROL

ON HEART DISEASE

The slow action of alpha tocopherol on heart disease is peculiar to that drug. If the cardiac patient begins on a full dose he will see no results for five to ten days and often no really definite and measurable improvement for three to four weeks. When, as often happens, he must begin on a small dose and increase it only very gradually, he will see no results until this period of time has elasped after reaching an effective dosage level. Fortunately, the slowness with which alpha tocopherol acts is coupled with a most desirable property—namely, that the improvement, once begun, continues for many months once the correct dose had been reached and provided that there are no complicating factors such as hypertension and hyperthyroidism (an overactive thyroid gland).

By contrast, alpha tocopherol usually acts rapidly in cases of acute phlebitis (leg clots), acute glomerulonephritis (Bright's disease) and the several diseases of the extremities seen in any peripheral

vascular clinic. We rarely see an acute glomerulonephritis or an acute phlebitis that does not show
great improvement within two weeks. Some cases of
acute rheumatic fever yield just as rapidly. There are
two reasons for the faster benefit achieved in treatment of these latter diseases. The first is that the
specific properties which accomplish this rapid
resolution are not those which play the major role in
the heart cases. In acute phlebitis and nephritis, for
example, the ability of the drug to resolve a thrombosis and to restore normal capillary permeability
are respectively responsible for rapid recovery,
while in most heart cases the specific actions of
greatest value are oxygen conservation and clot prevention (in contrast to clot resolution).

The second factor is the difference in the blood
supply reaching the heart (and brain) from that
found elsewhere in the body. While the structure of
the arteries and their branches is exactly the same
in all locations, there are fewer communicating
branches between the main vessels in the case of the
heart and the brain. Therefore, alpha tocopherol
reaches the individual cells of the heart and brain
less adequately than in the legs, for example, if damaged circulation is in process of restoration.

In heart disease alpha tocopherol is slow to act,
let us emphasize, but its beneficial effects are continuous. Less than the proper dose is ineffective. Too
much can be given, as we have so often emphasized,
notably in chronic rheumatic heart disease or with
hypertension. Diseases of veins respond to vitamin E
more readily than diseases of arteries for obvious
reasons.

Chapter 17

CONCURRENT PROBLEMS

IN VITAMIN E THERAPY

During the first *week* of treatment with vitamin E, diabetic patients should be especially alert for the occurrence of an overdose of insulin. Perhaps sugar should be present in the urine once a day in these patients. Otherwise the dose of insulin may be too great and should be reduced accordingly.

Thyroid deficiency (hypothyroidism) is very common. In doubtful cases a small daily dose, perhaps one-half grain of thyroid extract, is suggested. Give on rising in the morning. Increase every three weeks until signs of overdosage occur, such as elevated pulse rate, sweating, breathlessness, or tremor. Then revert to the dose found most suitable. Use least in summer and most in spring. We believe thyroid function tests are often misleading, rarely accurate, and generally unnecessary. This is a practical, if somewhat heretical view.

Hyperthyroid patients may not tolerate vitamin E. This is true even after surgical correction.

Dental infection can be important in heart patients. Any dental work should be preceded and followed by an adequate dose of a suitable antibiotic.

For a similar reason, even an apparently insignificant cold or flu, especially with cough, may be the cause of a serious setback. Keep the patient in bed until the temperature has been normal for several days.

Smoking never helps. In moderation it may do little harm, but it should be stopped, not merely decreased, when there is any evidence of congestive failure (fluid in lungs, congestion in liver, or swelling of the ankles), or especially in vascular disease of the extremities (such as Buerger's disease, for example, or hardened arteries). It induces vascular spasm, and that is what these people have to fear most. Vitamin E relaxes and dilates capillaries. Tobacco closes them. If they compete with each other, tobacco will win.

Alcohol is not advocated for heart disease by up-to-date doctors. It probably never helps the basic condition but may make the patient "feel better." It is dangerous to many patients who consistently take the maximum dosage, i.e., one or two ounces at a time, once or twice a day, with at least a four-hour interval between. Such patients may not be able to tell when they have begun to run into important symptoms of trouble—and this is a real danger, obviously. It may dilate skin vessels, but this is generally unhelpful and may do harm by robbing the deeper circulation. Recent studies indicate that actually alcohol depresses the heart muscle and is especially dangerous for patients in congestive failure.

Weight reduction should be carried to a reasonable level only. This can be done if excess weight has been caused by overeating. Reduction of overweight is difficult when associated with a family predisposition or beyond the age of fifty. Some people, large by reason of heavy bone and muscle structure, are not so much overweight as first impressions would suggest. No one should reduce below the weight at which they feel in best health. The lowest weight attainable by reasonable measures is advised. Appetite-limiting preparations may be used along with alpha tocopherol. Some people gain as much as fifteen pounds after starting vitamin E. Perhaps an improved sense of well-being induces heartier appetite. Diet-watching will soon correct this.

Test for Improvement: An exertion test should be carried out regularly after the patient has been on of an acute coronary attack. A moderately brisk walk vided that this is at least eight weeks from the time of an actue coronary attack. A moderately brisk walk on a level street is the best test. See how much distance can be covered before any of the symptoms of heart strain as described above develop. Record observations in a diary, because they are easily forgotten. Repeat this once a month and note any change. Activity which anyone may undertake at any and all times is that which good judgment will permit. Avoid any over-exertion which brings on symptoms of heart embarrassment. It is important to learn the limits of capacity. Above all, the patient should not do foolish things. Pushing a lawnmower seems to be a surprisingly common form of overexertion. Don't shovel snow or push a car. It isn't worth it.

Abdominal pain and tenderness in pregnancy is always alarming, particularly to a new mother-to-be. Doctors may carelessly say it is due to "stretch marks" or "adhesions" rather than progress to a more accurate diagnosis. That tender uterus (not abdomen, but *uterus*) means that placental detachment is imminent. The villi are losing their grip and often bleed. This is an indication of the need for large doses of alpha tocopherol. It is a timely specific and may prevent disaster.

Appendicitis is probably always *acute*, leaves one worse on flexing or on raising the leg, carries a 99.4 fever, has an increased white blood count and sedimentation rate. It hurts to stamp the foot or walk. Local rigidity over the right lower abdomen is found. Pain is often on both sides but much more evident on the right. Vitamin E has no effect on appendicitis.

Chapter 18

ALPHA TOCOPHEROL

FOR THE AGED

In the United States alone there are now over 13,000,000 people older than sixty-five. Two-thirds of these have an income averaging less than $1,000 per year, which means that insufficient food, insufficient care, and inadequate medical attention complicate the problems always attendant on the aging process. In Canada there are more than 1,000,000 persons over sixty-five. Comparable figures might apply to many another country. The problem is world-wide. Social and economic factors bear on these patients differently than on younger age groups. The problem is not only to alleviate what diseases the old have, but also to prevent an accumulation of disabilities among them.

The relative control of the infections has left cardiovascular and other deteriorations as the major problem of the elderly. Coronary disease and hypertensive arteriosclerotic heart disease head the list of

these. Hypertension affects more than one-third of
males over sixty. There is actually at the moment a
lesser expectancy of life among Americans sixty
years old and older than there was a hundred years
ago. It is the increase in heart disease which is
mainly responsible. For example, in Canada in the
decade 1941-50, deaths from heart disease increased
by 45 percent but the population by only 30 percent.
Most of the so-called increase of life expectancy is an
increase in the first third of the life span.

Arteriosclerotic changes of the brain are common, as everyone knows. This is the "dotage" of old
age. Those who display the worst symptoms, however, are often those who are also unsettled by fear,
insecurity and stress. Apoplexy may ensue, or
memory loss and mental changes, outbursts of unrea-
sonable anger and such. "Death often takes little
bites," says Dr. Alvarez of these people, and it may
take ten to twenty years to finish the task so gently
and insidiously begun.

Alpha tocopherol plays a valuable role in these
cases. We believe, of course, that it should be used in
association with all other helpful agents, for there
may be a multiple vitamin or other food deficiency in
poorly nourished old people. For example, they may
be anemic, in which case they may need iron for a
time. The alpha tocopherol should all be taken at
bedtime and any iron on rising. This separates them
in the stomach, for iron seems to knock out alpha tocopherol when they are taken by mouth simulta-
neously. Avoid dividing the tocopherol dose.

Alpha tocopherol is the most important precau-
tionary measure against strokes that one can suggest.

It helps to prevent clots forming in all blood vessels, and, of course, a clot in a vessel in the brain is what a stroke usually is. The aging hypertensive has this danger continually hanging overhead. Alpha tocopherol is some insurance against future strokes in the patient who has already experienced one—and everyone knows that these tend to repeat just as do coronary attacks. It often improves the damage in persons who have already had a stroke, but the degree of recovery is always unpredictable. It can be slow or minimal or marked. Certainly it demands a good and prolonged trial.

Alpha tocopherol salvages a good deal of the kidney function which is so frequently impaired in the elderly. Little else is helpful. Urinary frequency in the aged may be due to an enlarged prostate gland. The occasional man reports some small benefit to that condition when taking alpha tocopherol.

It is especially valuable for degenerative skin conditions in the genital area and anus, particularly in women. (*See* index.) This can be one of the most trying problems of the elderly. Restoration of skin circulation, something alpha tocopherol achieves best, may decrease itching or some types of dermatitis elsewhere on the body. Alpha tocopherol is taken in capsules or tablets orally, and tocopherol ointment is applied locally, or the ointment only is used.

Failing eyesight is occasionally helped, especially that caused by arteriosclerotic changes at the back of the eye, or, very rarely, cataract. (*See* index.)

High blood pressure may fall when alpha tocopherol is administered. It must be given cautiously,

and obviously by a physician, as we have stressed
before. (*See* index.) But it is quite effective in the
occasional patient, particularly when given in association with other antihypertensive agents.

The occasional bronchitic or asthmatic has developed a good deal of secondary heart muscle damage. This alpha tocopherol can help, although it
seems to have no effect upon the bronchitis itself.

But it is in heart disease in the aged that alpha
tocopherol is so uniquely valuable. No other agent
has such a beneficent effect upon heart muscle, and it
is the heart muscle that begins to fail at this period,
whether the primary injury was in the coronary circulation, due to thickening of the vessel wall, or associated with old rheumatic heart damage. It helps the
heart in failure, or the heart about to fail, although,
of course, other classical drugs may be needed as
well—digitalis or a diuretic, for example.

It enables damaged tissues to survive better on
less oxygen uptake. No other agent is as helpful in
this respect. Perhaps the tissues will do as well as
normally on an oxygen intake reduced by as much as
20 or more percent. It is nearly analogous to putting
a patient into an oxygen tent, where he probably actually gets an extra 30 percent of oxygen into his
bloodstream. The patient feels better and is better.

Alpha tocopherol tends to reduce the danger of
coronary clots in patients already showing hardened
coronary vessels and therefore suffering from angina.

It reduces or removes the leg cramps found in
elderly people whose leg circulation is greatly impaired. (*See* index.) Thus many an old person finally
gets a night's sleep once more. And is in much less

apprehension of gangrene realizing how often that ensues after a neglected arteriosclerosis of the leg vessels.

All in all, no other therapeutic agent has more, or as much, to offer the aging patient, particularly the one who already has ominous cardiovascular clouds on the horizon.

Chapter 19

HARDENING OF THE ARTERIES

(*Arteriosclerosis*)

Hardening of the arteries is a patchy but generalized disease very common in the elderly. Indeed, it has been popularly but incorrectly supposed to be a necessary and invariable concomitant of old age. Now we know that evidences of it appear early, perhaps much earlier in our day than in former decades, and certainly much earlier in our race and country than in many other races and countries. Seventy-seven percent of 300 American soldiers killed in Korea at an average age of twenty-two years were found to have this type of change in their coronary arteries—in contrast to their peers in the Korean army who had no evidence of previous cardiovascular disease.

Lengths of arteries, perhaps considerable stretches of them, develop thickening in the wall, usually just under their linings. These vessels degenerate until they may even calcify; thus so-called "pipe-stem" arteries develop. The bore of the vessel taking blood into the area involved decreases correspondingly and local tissues are starved. If the area is the brain, "senility," or dotage, may ensue—perhaps merely a change of character or loss of memory. If it is the heart that is involved, one may develop pain (angina) on only slight exertion, or perhaps an increased tendency to blood clotting (thrombosis). If it is the muscles, let us say the leg muscles, they can do less work without pausing for recuperation. Hence cramps develop on walking, or when the blood flow slows down in bed at night. Then the elderly patient must get up, walk around or hang his legs down as if he had Buerger's disease (see index)—as this condition is so frequently and carelessly miscalled. "Restless legs" (systremma) can prevent sleep.

The condition is slowly progressive, and becomes one of the most serious menaces in old age. The patient slowly slides into increasing disability, great pain or even gangrene. Most amputations in the elderly are to be ascribed to this disease. It plays a large role in high blood pressure, for it takes a greater head of pressure to force blood through such clogged, "limed-up" arteries. It plays a large role in strokes, where tiny brittle vessels in the brain may burst or clot. Its importance need not be stressed further.

Treatment has always been cursory or deceptive. No way to prevent the disease has been proposed until recent studies on cholesterol metabolism have suggested restriction of cholesterol-containing foods or fats in the diet. Some doubt of the efficacy of such diets has developed, especially since all such dietary regimes are instituted too late, after the disease has been operative for years and has already done its worst damage, and because such diets must be adhered to ever afterward. The principal measures in treatment have hitherto been aimed at avoiding injury to jeopardized tissues, reduction of any strenous activity to enable the incapacitated body to live within its elderly, narrow limits, and finally encouraging a move to hotter latitudes where damage by cold is less common.

Many vasodilating (vessel opening) drugs have been advocated, as for Buerger's disease. These have been disappointing. Sympathectomy has also been widely tried, a major surgical effort, resulting in transient and often inadequate benefit. Often amputation or multiple amputations are the final outcome, unless apoplexy cuts the story short.

Alpha tocopherol is very helpful in these patients if it is used in time, before irreparable damage has occurred. There must always be something to rescue if any therapeutic measure is to demonstrate what it can do. Even for gangrenous patients it offers hope, however. It may save what is left. It may delimit the gangrenous area and prevent its spread. It may prevent amputation.

Huge doses are needed and must be maintained for life. One of the first signs of improvement is the loss of night pain in the extremities, then decreased distress on walking, or the ability to cover a greater distance before being forced to stop to recover from the pain walking induces (claudication). Increased heat in the cold, emaciated extremities, a better color in the reddened, purplish feet, growth of nails, better cold tolerance, greater energy may ensue. However, in patients whose minds have deteriorated, no mental improvement can be anticipated, unfortunately. This point should be stressed. *When brain tissue has degenerated it cannot be restored. Such damage is permanent.*

There is occasionally, as in cases of Buerger's disease, severe, increased pain in the extremities as treatment begins. This is a good sign, due to the restoration of circulation in numb tissues. This resembles a frozen foot thawing out. It is hard to differentiate this pain from that felt in tissues dying from lack of circulation, however. Often only time can decide the source of the pain.

Tobacco should be forbidden to these patients. It produces vascular spasm in their peripheral arteries, and that adds insult to already far-advanced injury. These vessels are already partially closed; why close them further if one hopes to rescue the tissues they supply? The usual therapeutic measures have a place as well, of course—avoidance of cold, injury, ill-fitting shoes, and so on.

Chapter 20

VITAMIN E IN STROKES

These were touched upon briefly in Chapter 9. However, they are so common, so disabling not only to patients but to their families, and have such a tendency to recur, that perhaps more extended mention is justified.

A stroke can be major or minor. It can range all the way from the sudden fatal hemorrhage into and through the brain that is not too common, to the much commoner partial apoplexies. These latter can be very transient, even frequent, may cause no more than temporary weakness of a hand or the face or a foot, or can advance slowly and inexorably from very mild beginnings, and end in prolonged invalidism or in a quick fatality. The mild, transient strokes are probably due to spasm of the cerebral vessels or emboli, the severe and drastic ones to clots in vessels at the base of the brain.

They all tend to recur if the patient survives his initial attack. They are usually associated with high blood pressure and hardening of the arteries. They may leave a good deal of residual paralysis and weakness or merely "childish" character changes, gradual loss of memory and the higher mental powers. Death chews at these people, playing cat-and-mouse with them.

The prevention of hardening of the arteries is imperfectly understood. Diet may be a large factor in its causation, especially over-indulgence in animal fats. The prevention and treatment of hypertension is more effective of late, and no doubt would be still better if alpha tocopherol were used for more cases of incipient nephritis and for more pregnancy toxemias. But alpha tocopherol is most valuable here in its power to treat and prevent thrombosis or clotting in the damaged blood vessels. No other therapy has its unique qualities.

Even long after a stroke, alpha tocopherol sometimes seems to improve the palsy noticeably. More often it fails, for the damage has been irreparable. But its occasional success justifies its trial. And it is the only insurance against further attacks of clotting. Unfortunately, vitamin E never or only very rarely helps damage to brain function and personal character.

We believe all those who have hypertension and fear a stroke, all those who have had one and fear the usual recurrence, and all those who have residual paralysis after apoplexy, should be given alpha tocopherol. What else can one do? No one can suggest a good alternative. This is not to minimize the value of hypotensive drugs—merely to add to the doctor's kit the most useful agent he has yet found when he faces these distressed patients.

Chapter 21

VARICOSE VEINS AND

VARICOSE DERMATITIS

For years we refused to believe that alpha tocopherol could help varicose veins, despite a multitude of testimony from our patients. Now we believe it is worth trying, especially since alternative surgical measures ultimately give such poor results.

The mechanism appears to involve the fact that there are two sets of veins in the leg. The deep set we do not see. It normally returns about 85 percent of the blood flow from the foot. The other 15 percent comes back in the superficial veins that we recognize. The deep set is often blocked partially or nearly completely by old, unrecognized thrombi (clots) following a fracture, difficult childbirth or an operation where no such sequel was suspected. Deep blockage puts a greater strain on the superficial vessels. They dilate and twist and distend under the added burden. We say they become "varicose veins."

What has alpha tocopherol to offer? Its effect on

acute thrombosis is unique. Even old and chronic venous obstructions may sometimes—all too rarely— seem to resolve under its beneficial influence. Much more often, one suspects, it opens up multiple detours about the sites of venous obstruction and subtracts from the chronic burden on the overtaxed superficial veins. The latter shrink, become less congested and painful, the foot shows less swelling, and the patient is impressed by her relief. The leg does not go on to ulceration, collagenosis and increasing pain.

Certainly a brief trial of alpha tocopherol is worthwhile for troublesome varicose veins. In two months' time it should be obvious if it has anything to offer.

We no longer suggest injection of veins, or even ligations or stripping. No matter how carefully and thoroughly these are done, the frequent sequel is relief for twelve to eighteen months, then development of a new set of varicose veins to replace the old ones. *Such operations cannot reach and can do nothing for obstruction in the deep set of veins, which is the fundamental fault.* Certainly it is folly to operate on a leg that does not experience relief from the preliminary use of an elastic stocking. If the latter is not *obviously* helpful (it can make the leg more painful) it suggests strongly that closing the superficial set by elastic pressure or operation must only force more backflow on the deep set of veins which cannot handle it. Try the elastic stocking test, therefore, before any operation. Then do not have the operation. Few surgical measures are as disappointing—or as common! We very, very seldom advise one.

Varicose eczema is a common complication of varicosities in the leg. It can be chronic, very itchy, even weeping. It is often secondarily infected, crusted over, foul and malodorous, and may necessitate unsightly, stained bandages for many years on end, prevent walking, and be a constant and severe handicap.

It often responds well to alpha tocopherol, especially in ointment form. Many people find the ointment too irritating and must dilute it with vaseline, Nivea Creme, or some such bland ointment until its strength is halved or cut to one third. When it can be tolerated it is very helpful. When possible, alpha tocopherol should also be taken orally at the same time, of course.

One must be cautious here about producing generalized or far distant rashes as treatment is begun on any large area of eczema. For some unknown reason the whole body may react to our endeavors to treat a local area, and the same type of rash (called an "id" rash) may appear on the face, neck, arms, or elsewhere. That means "slow down," and treat less intensively, one small area at a time. Sometimes some other less irritating preparation of alpha tocopherol must be substituted for the type that has caused this upset.

Chapter 22

BLOOD CLOTS IN THE VEINS

(*Thrombosis, Phlebitis*)

Clots in the veins, often secondarily infected, often unrecognized, are all too common following fractures, childbirth or operation, notably such operations as those for hernia or appendicitis, or those performed on organs in the female pelvis. These are not only temporarily disabling, but they tend to promote chronic disability, with swollen, tender, painful legs hindering locomotion for years. Portions of fresh clots occasionally break loose into the circulation (embolism) and block off portions of the lung or brain, occasionally causing sudden death. The number of these cases appears to be on the increase, and the death and disability so produced have become major threats.

The popular agents used by medical men to date have been the so-called anticoagulants, drugs which hinder further blood clotting but do little or nothing to dissolve existing clots or provide detours around

plugged veins. They are dangerous, too—so dangerous that it is questionable if they have any place at
all in prolonged medical treatment. Indeed, there is a
good deal of medical debate on this issue at the moment.

What *is* the rationale for the anticoagulants?
What happens to the man who needs emergency surgery and is rendered inoperable by the fact that anti-
coagulant therapy has made him a hemophiliac? The
problem in the first place was not that his blood con-
gealed too fast, anyway. Although it is the treatment
of choice, it is by no means the safest or the best
treatment.

Alpha tocopherol is a happier answer and a safer
one. In large doses it not only prevents clots from
spreading, but it often melts them away rapidly, provides collateral circulation around the obstructed
vessels, and seems to prevent clots breaking loose as
emboli. Its effect upon fresh thrombosis or venous
clotting is truly amazing. Even the chronic case is occasionally helped, something that no other agent can
achieve. The probable mechanism here is the same as
in varicose veins; by-passes are developed around
old obstructions permitting a more normal circulation, less pain and swelling, and then allowing more
walking.

Moreover alpha tocopherol can prevent a recurrence, something that may develop even many years
after an acute attack. It is equally useful to prevent
initial attacks of clotting after operations or childbirth. Perhaps it should be used routinely in such
cases and in this way could end one of the most troublesome vascular conditions commonly encountered.

Some hospitals about the world have already begun to use it as a routine, postoperative preventive measure. (Professor Alton Ochsner, for example).[12]

We suspect that the patient who has had one or more attacks of thrombosis should always take some alpha tocopherol thereafter for the prevention of recurrence. A chance blow, a kick by a child, bumping a chair, even influenza can cause a phlebitis to flare up seven to twenty years after the initial attack. Presumably a residual lesion has slumbered in the affected vein all that time. If such a recurrence does appear in a patient already taking a small prophylactic dose of alpha tocopherol all she has to do is increase the dosage of alpha tocopherol at once, and the recurrence will be headed off almost before it has attained clear recognition.

That indolent ulcers often develop on the basis of a chronic phlebitis which induces stasis in the circulation of the leg has long been known. Many such ulcers heal and will remain healed on alpha tocopherol treatment, presumably because of better oxygenation of the tissues involved, but also, of course, because of the improved local circulation concurrently induced. In the collagenosis frequently associated with such chronic ulceration the alpha tocopherol is unable to induce resolution, but can limit the spread of the thickened, painful, discolored, leathery area. (See index.)

In the typical acute phlebitis or thrombosis one must administer enough alpha tocopherol to do the job. The response is so rapid and dramatic on the proper dose that if no such good result develops within three to five days' time one should merely increase it to find the dose that will win conspicuously and quickly.

We leave all such patients free to move about during treatment. We put none to bed.

Phlebitis, occurring particularly after fractures treated in casts, is so common and so often unrecognized that one should stress the point here. Phlebitis causes tenderness along the course of veins, (especially on squeezing the leg from side to side), swelling of the foot or leg, even redness and increased skin heat. Physicians should be more alert than they are to detect this complication, especially after fracture casts have been on for some time or have been taken off after long immobilization. The best single sign is tenderness of the leg on lateral compression. But even so, 50 percent of cases of deep venous thrombosis show no physical signs, it is now held. I personally disagree with this figure and feel a proper examination of endangered legs would find many more cases now being missed.

Chapter 23

VITAMIN E OINTMENT

It has long been known that alpha tocopherol can be absorbed through the skin and mucous membranes, but medical and lay people generally tend to think of it as an oral medication. Its local application should not be neglected.

It is valuable in the myositis-fibrositis-myalgia group of complaints. These are commonly referred to by the man on the street as "muscular rheumatism." There it may be applied once or twice daily, with gentle massage for at least ten minutes, and followed by local heat such as a heating pad or hot water bottle.

It is very useful when applied to chronic ulcers or eczemas, notably those associated with varicose veins. Such patients should also take it by mouth, of course. Many people find it irritating when applied to skin lesions, and must dilute it by at least half with vaseline, Nivea Creme, or some other such base.

It accelerates the healing of fresh wounds as well, and is particularly valuable for wounds on the face, where stitches may be almost as disfiguring as the laceration they were meant to repair. Healing of any raw area is a race between the granulation tissue growing upward from the depths of the wound and the skin coming in from its edges. If one uses alpha tocopherol, the latter wins, and the resultant scar is pliable, level with adjacent skin, flexible, and uncontracted. With every type of healing the resultant scar tends to contract and pucker up with the passage of time. Hence the tendency of surgeons to do skin grafts, especially near joints. Much of this grafting is no longer needed since the introduction of tocopherol, for vitamin E produces an uncontracted kind of scar never seen before, and nearly ideal.

It is the local treatment par excellence for burns, whether minor household burns, sunburn, chemical burns, or graver injuries. All deep burns should be treated topically with vitamin E ointment and combined with vitamin E capsules taken orally. Once it has been used for a burn, no one will ever neglect its use again. It has become obvious that it has no equal in this sphere of healing.

At the moment, radiation burns constitute one of the greatest menaces to mankind. X-ray burns and radium burns respond better to alpha tocopherol than to any other agents we know. We feel that the existence of such a cheap, simple, self-applicable, concentrated medical agent is of supreme importance to modern populations, in time of war especially.

Vitamin E ointment probably will prove useful in many skin diseases where its value has not yet

been explored. We suspect it may often help sebor-
rhea and pityriasis, for example. Psoriasis is rarely
helped, unfortunately.

Certainly it is often useful for rheumatoid arthritis of the small joints of the hands. However, it
very rarely seems to be helpful for arthritis of larger
joints. Muscle bruises and strains may respond to its
local application.

Before finishing this chapter let me stress again
the value of vitamin E ointment for burns over
knuckles and of the cornea. Help is obviously direly
needed here and yet so inadequate as we now handle
such emergencies. Poor results ruin a life, medically
and socially. *Try E for burns*. It is wonderfully helpful.

Chapter 24

VASCULAR COMPLICATIONS

OF DIABETES

On the twenty-fifth anniversary of the discovery of insulin, and in the years since, there has been a great deal of investigation of patients thoroughly treated with dietary restriction and insulin for the quarter century. Nearly every investigator has come up with the rather appalling finding that there seem to be two phases of diabetes. One is high blood sugar, recognized so long as being the outstanding derangement in body function, and the other is vascular degeneration, which assaults the body's whole vascular tree, notably the eyes. The discouraging point has been made by many workers that the best insulin and dietary treatment seems to have little effect in retarding these vascular degenerations. The result is that even the young diabetic on ordinary treatment has become an old man in twenty-five years' time, who may display intense hardening of the arteries of the extremities by then, even gangrene, and is almost

sure to have deterioration of eyesight or cataract.
Changes in the heart and kidneys are very common
also, although not quite so obvious.

Into this situation came vitamin E. Of course, it
seemed to many diabetic specialists to be a far cry
from the use of this agent for the prevention of miscarriage, or for burns, or for heart pain, to its application in diabetes. But, independently, Butturini[13] of
Italy and the Shute brothers each recorded observations indicating that the use of alpha tocopherol in
diabetes was of real value. Both groups of workers,
and others who have confirmed these observations
since, have pointed out that some diabetics require
less insulin after taking alpha tocopherol. They may
develop insulin reactions from doses of the latter
they have long tolerated. These must be watched for.
Most diabetics, however, especially youngsters, remain on about the same dosage as before they took
alpha tocopherol. All diabetics taking alpha tocopherol for the first time should carry candy in their
pocket for the first three days.

The most spectacular results are achieved in
vascular degenerations of the extremities, the use of
alpha tocopherol preserving many a foot and leg
threatened with amputation on account of diabetic
gangrene or intractable discharging sinuses. Many
photographs of such lesions are in the possession of
the Shute Institute for Medical Research, and some
of these have been demonstrated at meetings of the
British Medical Association, the Canadian Medical
Association, the Ontario Medical Association, the
American Osteopathic Association, and other such
major medical meetings. They are among the most

dramatic examples of the power of alpha tocopherol to salvage situations that are otherwise hopeless.

We think that the time will soon come when every diabetic, as soon as his condition is recognized, will realize that his treatment is inadequate unless he takes alpha tocopherol as well as using the traditional insulin with dietary restrictions or the now controversial oral hypoglycemic agents introduced in recent years into diabetic management. This new point of view is of especial significance for the juvenile diabetic, who otherwise progresses steadily downhill and becomes prematurely aged.

Is it any wonder that diabetes ranks fifth on the list of causes of death more than fifty years after the discovery of insulin? We say that alpha tocopherol plugged the leak in the insulin boat.

Chapter 25

SMALL AREAS OF GANGRENE

Small areas of gangrene in the extremities do not necessarily demand amputation nowadays, particularly amputation high in the leg. Surgeons generally tend to suggest such amputations, but their opinions must now be reconsidered. It is alpha tocopherol that has altered this situation. Other treatment may continue to be used at the same time, and all the usual and obvious precautions must be maintained. But alpha tocopherol is the unrivaled prime curative agent.

Such gangrenous areas may develop for many reasons, the commonest being arteriosclerosis, diabetes and Buerger's disease. They arise whenever the blood supply to these areas becomes so impaired that the tissues cannot survive, therefore die and turn black. Once tissues have died they never can be revived, but the gangrene can theoretically be prevented from spreading if sufficient circulation is restored to adjacent tissues and the dead tissues can be walled off and detached. Then only local amputations of small areas may be demanded, or nature herself may spontaneously amputate small dead areas.

Experience shows that many such areas of gangrene can be delimited if alpha tocopherol is administered in huge doses. The best results are achieved in diabetics, fully 25 percent of these eventually being able to reduce their insulin dosage; the next best appear in Buerger's disease, and the poorest in hardening of the arteries.

This is due partly to the development of collateral circulation about the blocked vessels, and partly to the increased ability of the local tissues to utilize oxygen under this treatment. Such tissues can now survive with a lesser blood supply than before. They obviously need this increased survival margin desperately. Only alpha tocopherol can supply it readily and sustain it for a long time.

Of course, alpha tocopherol should be administered to every diabetic or arteriosclerotic long *before* gangrene develops. One wonders why people wait so long when every other treatment has failed before trying such a helpful agent as alpha tocopherol. But even after small areas have become frankly gangrenous the situation need not always be thought hopeless. Alpha tocopherol should always be tried. A decrease of local pain, increased heat in the extremities, perhaps the ability to sleep throughout the night with the leg up in bed, even early signs of separation of the gangrenous area, are the first evidences of improvement. The results will often amaze both patient and physician.

However, pain alone can be intolerable and cut short any prolonged trial of tocopherol therapy. A patient can endure only so much pain before becoming addicted to narcotics or so ill that amputation becomes a necessary work of mercy. And tocopherol may worsen the pain in a leg deprived of adequate circulation, analogous to the increased pain on thawing a cold hand. The patient may be unable to tolerate this, in which case treatment can be stopped, or may be given more gradually from an initial lower level, or may be forced at a high level of dosage in order to cut short the torture of the therapeutic effort.

After healing, the alpha tocopherol must be maintained indefinitely, for the rescued tissues need to have their circulation and oxygen supply bolstered up continually. The other leg needs this especially, for so often it soon follows suit unless such precautions are taken.

One of the puzzling situations in surgery is the tendency we have, as physicians, to look at one extremity, the one involved, only. We should remember that arteriosclerosis or diabetes affects one leg as severely as the other. One leg is just a step behind its mate. When treatment of the involved leg is completed either with success or failure, our task is unfinished, for *we must watch and treat the other leg.* A point so obvious should not need to be made, even to those not medically trained. The truth is that this warning is rarely if ever heeded!

Our information is insufficient on what alpha tocopherol has to offer such related conditions as frozen extremities, "immersion foot," "trench foot," and such—but tocopherol therapy justifies trial there as well.

Chapter 26

INDOLENT LEG ULCERS

Chronic leg ulcers have been ascribed to varicose veins, injury of various kinds, or to plain "stasis" or stagnation. Chronic infection usually supervenes, and congestion can produce severe, burning, aching pain. Many of these heal slowly, then break down repeatedly, and may persist in this way for fifteen to twenty-five years. They become foul. Dirty bandages conceal them inside bulging stockings. Scar or collagenosis forms a broad band around them, perhaps girdling the leg. For years these embarrassed people limp along in pain, concealing their disease as well as they can.

Alpha tocopherol is the newest and most helpful agent in their treatment. Often it needs to be used in association with other classical measures such as heat, elevation in bed, antibiotics applied locally, perhaps after erosive agents able to eat away their overlying crusts have been applied. But it is the most helpful single item, and often wins by itself in the most persistent cases.

Here the ointment is very valuable. Many people find it too strong in its usual concentration, and must dilute it considerably with vaseline, eucerin ointment, or Nivea Creme if it burns or produces weeping. But a thin layer of ointment on gauze should be applied twice a day, if possible. Better still, one may leave the ulcer exposed, free of all dressings, and apply the ointment.

High dosages of alpha tocopherol by mouth at the same time are important. One watches for a fine whitish rim to develop around the ulcer, then for islands to develop throughout its area, then for the encroachment of peninsulas resembling spontaneous skin grafts.

Even after healing has occurred, alpha tocopherol should be continued for months or years in order to maintain local tissue oxygenation and circulation and so prevent the ulcers from recurring. Stopping treatment when the lesion heals is a constant source of disappointment to patients. They should remember that the cause usually persists. What produced the first ulcer can readily produce another. Each time one heals the area is damaged further, and scarring impedes local circulation and tissue oxygenation. Hence the need for taking alpha tocopherol long after healing has been completed.

Since the legs are so similar, there is a great tendency for ulcers and other leg lesions to become bilateral. This is especially true of the dense scarring of collagenosis. (See index.) It nearly always girdles one leg, then the other, unless its extension is prevented by an *adequate* dose of alpha tocopherol, whatever that dose may be. Nothing else that we know of can prevent the progression around one leg, then the other, until it becomes a sort of leather band around and above each ankle. Vitamin E cannot soften or reduce it, but it can prevent it from spreading and ulcerating, unless too badly injured.

Chapter 27

BUERGER'S DISEASE

This disease is a rather odd one. It is very rarely
seen in women. It has a predilection for younger
men, often those in their twenties or thirties, rarely
occurring in men over forty-five. It is asymmetrical,
for some strange reason usually attacking the feet before the hands, and one toe or one foot before the
others. In the end it tends to affect all four extremities.

It may show itself first as calf cramps or foot
cramps upon walking. These compel the sufferer to
rest until the cramp leaves; then he can go on again
for a short distance until the cramp returns. This
muscle cramp does not leave soreness afterward, unlike the cramp due to calcium deficiency and called te-
tany. Much later on these cramps develop at night,
preventing sleep, occasionally in bad cases forcing a
man to get up to walk about during the night or sit
up with his foot hanging over the edge of the bed.

Later on, gangrene supervenes. It may involve
only one toe or a portion of it, or several toes, or
larger areas of the foot. The extremity is very painful in the adjacent areas, scarcely permitting touch
or the weight of bed clothes. This process rapidly
spreads until it compels amputation of one, then of
another extremity. The severest cases may lose all
four over the course of a few years. Meantime the
suffering can be extreme.

The popular medical approach to this problem is
sympathectomy—cutting the so-called "sympathetic"
chain of nerves near the spinal column in the lower
back. This dilates the small twigs of the arteries of
the corresponding extremity and *for a time* restores
better circulation *in the skin*. The difficulty is that
this expensive, delicate, often severely shocking operation so often gives only very slight or no relief. Its
benefit may be largely confined to the skin. Then the
painful march of the gangrene resumes. Many vasodilating agents have been widely used, such as pris-
coline or raniacol. We have been disappointed in
these, as have most other workers. They, too, tend to
dilate skin vessels only, and in doing so may rob the
deep vessels.

Alpha tocopherol is much the most effective
agent yet tried. It is a vasodilator, an agent capable
of opening up very tiny blood vessels or capillaries.
It acts on deep tissues as well as skin. If used in time
it relieves night pain, pain on walking (claudication), and may stave off or delimit gangrene. It protects other areas of the extremities from the assault
of this dreadful disease. It protects the brain, heart
and kidneys which are often as involved as the legs,

although not so conspicuously. Such involvement should always be looked for, however.

Alpha tocopherol must be used in very high dosage, and used for the remainder of life, for these patients are always under risk as long as they live. Tobacco must be *absolutely* forbidden upon making the diagnosis. It is *not enough to cut down*. The patient is to be warned: it is a choice between *absolute abstinence* from tobacco and preserving the legs. Extremes of cold must be avoided. Naturally these people do better in warm latitudes.

We warn men beginning tocopherol treatment that they may experience severe initial pain in the foot or leg as new circulation develops in tissue previously almost devoid of circulation. This distress is difficult to differentiate from the pain felt by the patient earlier, before treatment was begun—but time will settle the point very quickly. Meantime the patient must be a patient patient.

What has been said earlier about the increased pain some men experience on tocopherol therapy should be re-emphasized here. One may need to begin at small dosage levels, perhaps a mere 200 I.U. daily, and increase slowly week by week to a more appropriate dosage because of the increased pain if large doses are initially administered. The patient may complain of formication ("worms" in his leg) at high initial dosage, perhaps due to little collateral vessels re-opening in his deep tissues. Formication disappears as he becomes able to tolerate big doses of vitamin E.

Chapter 28

BURNS

Alpha tocopherol is unrivaled in the treatment of burns, whether it is used in ointment form, or taken in capsule or tablet form orally, or in combined topical and oral form. This is as true of X-ray burns as of ordinary thermal or chemical burns.

The application of tocopherol ointment locally may be alternated with an antibiotic ointment if the wound surface has become infected. The former is soothing and soon relieves pain in the area. It should, of course, always be accompanied by the administration of large doses of alpha tocopherol by mouth.

The usual difficulty in burn healing is that the wound edges lose in the race against the granulation tissue growing up from the base to form scar. The result is a heaped up, disfiguring cicatrix, which tends to immobilize adjacent joints or to deform the area. Hence the need for skin grafting in so many burn cases. In any case healing is tedious, painful and costly by all the traditional methods surgeons use.

The wounds healed by alpha tocopherol therapy are level with the adjacent skin, flexible, and not contracted, which is almost unheard of in other burn treatment.

Even sunburn or chemical burns are well handled by alpha tocopherol.

It should be of unique value in the day of the atom and hydrogen bomb, for it is cheap, stable, not bulky, and can be self-applied.

Some people heal burns with heaped up, tender or itchy scars called keloids. The itching these create may be intolerable if the scarred tissue is extensive. Nothing seems to give such ease as tocopherol ointment, and the result is achieved very quickly.

Chapter 29

CERTAIN EYE DISEASES

The uses of alpha tocopherol in this field are not yet well explored. Certain conditions seem to respond occasionally, and others much oftener. For example, although the results in most cataracts are quite disappointing the odd case responds well. Dr. Wilfrid Shute had a cataractous dog which once again became able to kill rats after treatment. We have seen a few patients with choroiditis who were obviously helped. These are instances of the roles that alpha tocopherol may later be found to play in eye disease, for example in thrombosis of the central vein or retinal detachment. At the moment little is known of its place in such conditions.

But it has a definite place in the arteriosclerotic eye, where there are multiple small hemorrhages in the retina. There is good evidence that abnormal capillary permeability is decreased by the administration of alpha tocopherol. Thus further hemorrhages should be hindered. Moreover the increased local circulation should assist in the reabsorption of hemorrhages already present. Often one eye is much more involved than the other. The real problem is not only to restore the damaged eye but to protect its mate, whose importance has suddenly multiplied. Here is one of the most vital potential values of alpha tocopherol.

Opthalmologists we know well have told us of degeneration of the macula responding to oral alpha tocopherol. However, it may benefit one eye and not the other.

Dr. Wilfrid Shute has used the ointment or the oral capsules of oil successfully for corneal ulcers. He simply breaks a capsule (400 I.U.) and spills the oil in the open eye.

We suspect that opthalmologists have a fertile field for exploration here, notably in burns.

Chapter 30

KIDNEY DISEASE

(Glomerulonephritis)

This disease is rarer than formerly, although still not rare enough. It is characterized by the sudden appearance of albumin in the urine and swelling of the face, extremities, or body, sometimes accompanied by an elevation of blood pressure, rarely by obvious blood in the urine. It may follow an attack of scarlet fever, or acute tonsillitis, even a mild cold by ten to fourteen days. It may run an acute, rapidly fatal course, but often it tends to subside spontaneously after a few weeks or months. Many cases slumber on indefinitely and become chronic, occasionally with recurrences of more acute phases. Some cases are regarded as a kidney reaction to a streptococcus. It is usually treated with rest, dietary restriction and antibiotics, but is very imperfectly understood, and treatment is much more disappointing than the above summary of somewhat obvious complaints would lead one to expect. Medical men differ widely among

themselves about every aspect of this disease. It is
commonly assumed, however, that many a case of
hypertension or albuminuria (albumin in the urine)
in adult life may have begun with mild attacks of
kidney involvement of this type, and that better handling of the early attack could perhaps prevent much
high blood pressure later. There seems to be no true
correlation between the severity of the tonsillitis or
other upper respiratory disease and the onset of an
acute glomerulonephritis, or its failure to develop.
Perhaps only one or at most two strains of the streptococcus matter. This is one more reason to pay serious attention to even "ordinary" sore throats. They
may be precursors of hidden, mysterious assaults of
nephritis. The recent decrease in frequency of this
disease may perhaps be ascribed to better treatment
of acute sore throats with sulfa drugs or antibiotics.

Alpha tocopherol plays a wonderful role in the
acute cases. It far surpasses any other agent so far
used. It may smother the early phase as water smoth-
ers a fire. Doses should be large, and other ordinary
precautions should be observed about handling tonsillitis or other attendant infection. There is real
hope, too early yet to state with any assurance, that
the rapid resolution of the acute phase of the disease
by alpha tocopherol may prevent many of the late or
chronic cases from developing, and thus may prevent
some hypertensions in later life.

Certainly alpha tocopherol should always be
tried as early as diagnosis has been made. It should
continue to be administered for months or years after clinical "cure" has developed.

Unfortunately, there is no reason to feel that

true "nephrosis" in children responds well to alpha tocopherol. This appears to be a different type of kidney disease. It is characterized by *huge* swelling, much albumin in the urine but no blood, and certain alterations in the ratio of blood protein fractions.

This disease deserves more attention than it has received. Kidney transplants can scarcely be the best answer. They are too tedious and distressing, alter the whole life style of a family as well as the patient himself, and at best are merely palliative.

Chapter 31

MISCARRIAGE AND PREMATURITY

Vitamin E first came into clinical use in 1932 when the Danish veterinarian, Philip Vogt-Moller, picked up the studies carried out ten years earlier at the University of California and Arkansas and used this substance for human miscarriage.[14] He reported that repeated miscarriages, technically called "habitual abortion," could be prevented by the administration of this vitamin to the pregnant woman. At that time a fresh ether-extracted wheat germ oil was its only source.

Many other workers confirmed his findings. But after 1938 a wave of medical skepticism came to the fore and a female sex hormone, progesterone, has almost replaced it in the years since. The latter now has encountered severe criticism in its turn and alpha tocopherol is probably due to return to wider use as the use of progesterone and progestogenic substances wanes.

The great difficulty in assessing such treatment derives from the fact that many miscarriages cannot possibly be stopped by any measure the doctor uses. They are pregnancies in which the embryo is imperfectly formed or sits and exists upon an inadequate afterbirth. It is reliably reported now that only 15 to 20 percent of those pregnancies that threaten to miscarry and do not respond to simple bed rest are capable of salvage. And bed rest alone appears to rescue some 30 to 40 percent. What agent is most effective in saving the precarious but small group indicated above?

We feel that alpha tocopherol is that agent. It is increasingly effective, of course, for those threatened terminations that reveal themselves as pregnancy continues. Thus it is better able to rescue the seven-months child than the five months, for example, or the five-months foetus than the two-months embryo. But it is always worthy of trial, in large doses, combined with bed rest, cessation of intercourse, and the usual older medical measures.

Not only should it be tried if miscarriage threatens. It should be given long before that, indeed as soon as pregnancy is recognized. The great difficulty of waiting to see if it is needed to ward off trouble is that miscarriage can threaten very suddenly, apparently out of a clear sky. Before any alpha tocopherol that is administered has had time to take effect the embryo may have been fatally jeopardized or even expelled. We feel, therefore, that every pregnant woman should be given alpha tocopherol in proper dosage from the time of first recognition of her pregnancy.

As we have said, alpha tocopherol seems to be able to rescue a considerable proportion of women who threaten to terminate their pregnancies too soon, the percentage rising as the period of gestation advances. Thus in the last two months of pregnancy, over 70 percent of precarious cases may be rescued, and a corresponding group of women may remain pregnant even after early rupture of their membranes and appreciable loss of the watery fluid which normally cushions the infant in the womb.

Occasionally women are told that it is unwise to preserve precarious pregnancies lest deformed children be born. The evidence for this point of view is very unsatisfactory. Every threatened pregnancy should be saved if it can be. Mothers carrying such pregnancies have very little reason to fear that they are thus jeopardizing the child.

Pregnant women should take vitamin E *until the baby comes,* unless they develop the elevation of blood pressure, albumin in the urine and swelling of the legs near term that is of the comparatively rare type apt to end in convulsions. The doctor must decide if there is danger of fits, and then he may decide to stop the vitamin E and administer an antagonistic substance, female sex hormone, in order to ward off this danger.

Being "well born" is an old phrase that has always been nearly meaningless. Now it no longer is. Many of the ills of pregnancy appear to be determined at the moment conception occurs. It is important that the best possible sperm (male cell) meets and fertilizes the best possible ovum (female cell or egg) at that moment. Since the egg appears to be inaccessible to medical treatment, this happy result is best assured by treating the husband. He should stop tobacco for at least several weeks before conception and he should be given a relatively small dose of alpha tocopherol (100 to 200 I.U. daily). This is especially important where previous pregnancies have had an unfortunate outcome—for example, have ended in a deformed child. The mother should take vitamin E as soon as she conceives, for the child is not formed completely until the twelfth week of pregnancy.

There is a condition where the child habitually dies in the womb just prior to delivery. Here, too, alpha tocopherol is indicated. It should probably be administered to the husband before further conceptions. It should certainly be given to the mother from conception *until delivery,* the dose being increased considerably at about the time when the earlier children perished.

Chapter 32

VITAMIN E IN STERILITY AND

HABITUAL MISCARRIAGE

Alpha tocopherol seems to have no influence on sterility in the human female.

But it has been shown to influence male germ cells (sperm) at least qualitatively. In this way it seems to be able to help couples where the wife habitually miscarries. If given to the sire before conception, and to the wife thereafter, her chances of carrying her child are materially enhanced. The man should be forbidden tobacco at the same time, if he uses it.

It is especially useful in those families where one or more structurally defective children have been born. The tendency for "anomalies," as these are called, to repeat is well known. It has been estimated, for example, that if one child in a family is thus defective at birth, the chances of another brother or sister being structurally defective are increased by seven times, or to about one in seven—

from the "norm" we have found (for our particular locality) of one in forty-five births. Great success has been reported where the sire in such families has been given alpha tocopherol *before all subsequent conceptions.* He should take vitamin E for at least three weeks before such later conceptions occur; in these families conceptions should not just "happen." They should be carefully planned and prepared for as indicated above.

When men have followed this advice and had normal children, they may relax the precautions noted above, feeling that they are no longer necessary. No greater mistake could be made. We have seen a good deal of tragedy ensue on such carelessness. Therefore, we strongly urge that these directions regarding alpha tocopherol and tobacco be observed before *all* subsequent conceptions in a family where one defective child has been born.

No problem in obstetrics is more poignant or more ignored than congenital defect in infants. A hare lip, or clubfoot or congenitally defective heart can ruin the outlook of a whole family, and increase the care needed to raise the child. The emotional stress on parents is indescribable. Alpha tocopherol should always be taken before any *future conceptions,* especially by the sire.

Chapter 33

MENSTRUAL PROBLEMS
AND OTHER DISEASES
PECULIAR TO WOMEN

Heavy or scanty menstrual periods are not influenced by alpha tocopherol—but women with painful periods often receive help if this agent is taken for several days before the flow begins.

One of the most generally recognized uses of alpha tocopherol is for hot flushes and headaches at the change of life (menopause). Female sex hormone is the agent generally used for menopausal complaints, but too often this causes vaginal bleeding or "spotting" which alarms the patient and her doctor; they may suspect cancer. Alpha tocopherol never induces such spotting and is never in any way involved either in accelerating the growth of cancers already present or in initiating them. There is some suspicion that estrogenic substances may. Alpha tocopherol is usually not as effective as the latter for hot flushes, but it is often helpful, and its safety factor is strongly in its favor. Once in a while *normal* menstrual periods may return for a time after it is administered. This should not be alarming. It is strictly a return toward normal, not an abnormality.

Moreover it is valuable for the itching of the external genitals so often found at this time of life, sometimes associated with local skin degenerations which are ugly, acutely painful and potentially dangerous. Very high dosage, perhaps continued for long periods of time, is demanded in the treatment of these vulvar degenerations, and four to six weeks usually elapse before a response to treatment first appears. Often such a condition is the first warning of diabetes, and there, too, alpha tocopherol is extremely valuable, both for diabetic vulvitis and for other complications of that disease. By the use of alpha tocopherol, X ray, local operations and all sorts of messy ointments applied locally may be obviated in most instances. Some women have local itching ascribed to discharge that persists long after the discharge has been cured. These women really have had two kinds of itching at once. Cure the one and the other comes to the fore. Alpha tocopherol may help these people too, relieving the type of itching which has been unjustifiably ascribed before to the discharge.

Not only the vulva but the anus may become itchy as the skin becomes senile at this critical time of life. Alpha tocopherol in ointment form locally, as well as taken by mouth in pill or capsule, is very helpful here. Men itch too, and are helped similarly.

Probably alpha tocopherol has no effect upon female sterility. It was originally called a "fertility" or sterility vitamin, but that name was given it by rat experimenters who used the term in a different sense than clinicians do.

Diffusely painful breasts are often helped by alpha tocopherol. Such breasts may contain tiny lumps or cysts (chronic mastitis). These are usually not worthy of worry if they show themselves in both breasts. (Remember breast cancer nearly always begins and long remains on one side only, and is not tender to the touch.) The ointment can be rubbed in, but alpha tocopherol should also be given by mouth. Relief is often surprisingly quick and complete. This could become one of the major uses of vitamin E, for chronic mastitis is common and frightening. There are too many operations for this condition.

It has even been suggested that women having small, asymptomatic "fibroid" tumors of the womb should take alpha tocopherol regularly and faithfully to hinder further growth of the tumors. These small tumors very rarely demand operation, contrary to former medical opinion. They have no undue tendency to become associated with cancer and can usually be almost ignored—apart from taking alpha tocopherol and having their future course followed by a gynecologist in case too much menstrual bleeding develops, notably "spotting."

Chapter 34

THE TOXEMIA OF PREGNANCY

THAT DOES NOT

PRODUCE CONVULSIONS

Many a pregnant woman in the last few months develops an undue gain of weight, swelling of the extremities, albumin in the urine and a rising blood
pressure. This is called "toxemia."

There are two main types. One is sudden in onset, severe from the first, and rapidly goes on to convulsions. This type is very dangerous to the mother
and may even be fatal.

It is to be differentiated from the type that is
about eight or nine times commoner, where the same
phenomena seem to appear much more deliberately
and gradually, with a hypertension not so marked,
perhaps more swelling than the other type of woman
displays, and yet no tendency to convulse. This patient's illness tends to kill her unborn child, usually
by separation of the afterbirth and this is often accompanied by severe pain in the womb and by
bleeding.

This latter type seems to be prevented or helped by alpha tocopherol. The best treatment is prevention, of course, and this is one reason we believe tocopherols should be given to *every* pregnant woman from the time she suspects a pregnancy. Larger doses are required as the so-called toxic symptoms become more severe. At any time toward the very end of pregnancy this type may suddenly alter to the severer, preconvulsive type. Then the skilled obstetrician quickly stops alpha tocopherol, which at this crisis can make his patient's condition worse, and changes to estrogen (female sex hormone) therapy.

Alpha tocopherol tends to anchor the afterbirth in the second and common type of toxemia, perhaps providing better local circulation in this organ, which is the basic circulatory and nutritive organ of the yet-unborn infant. It is widely believed that the afterbirth is the source of the toxins or other such agents which damage mother and child in these "toxic" states. Presumably an afterbirth kept from degenerating by an improved circulation is less apt to release such noxious agents. Increased oxygenation, too, must play a role, for the unborn child lives at levels of oxygen intake on which no adult could survive. These can readily drop to concentrations too low for the child. Giving alpha tocopherol is a precaution against such a catastrophe.

In the toxemia of this type alpha tocopherol should be given until delivery. It is useful after delivery in *both* types where any evidence of kidney damage or high blood pressure persists, for no agent is as helpful after such kidney damage as alpha tocopherol.

Chapter 35

SCAR TISSUE AND

COLLAGENOSIS

There is a condition known as Dupuytren's contracture, a scarring and contraction of the deep tissues of the palm which pull up the fingers into something resembling a claw. Usually the fourth and fifth fingers are more apt to be involved than the others. More rarely this clawing develops on the sole of the foot. It has always been treated surgically, although it tends to recur after operation. Alpha tocopherol relieves a percentage of such patients, in whole or in part, even after the scarring has existed for years. The result it provides seems to be comparable to that obtained by operation, however less than perfect and however variable.

There is a broad group of disease conditions often called "muscular rheumatism" for lack of a better term. We refer to such sore tissues as myalgia or myositis if muscle is principally involved, or even fibrositis if it is suspected that connective tissue fibers are more affected. Septic foci such as infected teeth or tonsils may be responsible, but often the disease persists after these have been removed. Then heat, together with the administration of alpha tocopherol, and, best of all, alpha tocopherol applied in ointment form and gently rubbed into the tender areas for ten-minute periods often seem very helpful. Certainly alpha tocopherol should be tried, in addition to the usual attempts to find the causative factors and eradicate them.

Collagenosis is a common condition, indeed. (*See* index.) It is the dense, discolored, leather-like scarring seen around so many chronic ulcers or in chronic phlebitis. The skin clings close to the bone and perhaps tightens about the leg, forcing the soft tissues of the calf to bulge out above. It is usually either bilateral or soon begins to involve both legs. At first it is pink or red; later it is usually purple or brown. It never seems to involve the thigh or the upper extremities. Sometimes it is exquisitely tender in the early months or years, slowly becoming numb as leather. Gradually it spreads out at the edges until it extends over the ankle and half way to the knee—rarely higher.

Until alpha tocopherol was used no other treatment for this condition seems to have evolved. And the latter in its turn does not heal or resolve the thickened tissues. *In the proper dosage,* however, and *as long as it is continued* it prevents the process from extending, or from attacking the corresponding part of the other leg. Large doses are needed—and *must be taken indefinitely.*

Chapter 36

VITAMIN E FOR ATHLETES

Athletes are using muscles under conditions of maximum stress, are pushing their heart and lung capabilities to the utmost, and are constantly seeking to get even more achievement out of their bodies. It is natural that where small margins make the difference between defeat and victory, or between mere winning and setting a record, the effect of such an agent as alpha tocopherol should be investigated.

The number of studies reported has been few, and we ourselves have no personal experience in the field. However, the late Mr. Lloyd Percival of Canada's Sports College has done a good deal of work in this field.[15]

Mr. Percival used large doses of concentrated tocopherols. He reported greater endurance, better "wind," an improved feeling of well-being generally. Champion performers developed out of mediocre athletes on this new regimen. Percival noted less accel-

eration of pulse on exertion in athletes taking E, also
a faster reversion to normal, sometimes more sweating, certainly less muscle fatigue and faster recovery
of ability to re-run a race.

A quotation from his report puts this succinctly:
"In another 'side' test members of the Toronto Track
Club were separated into two groups. Half were
given 'E' two weeks before the Canadian champion-
ship meet, half were not. The two groups were separated evenly in regard to talent and standing as
performers. The group given 'E' had a much better
performance in their meet than did those not on 'E.'
This was especially true in events from the '440' up!
Members on 'E' broke 9 Canadian records and 2
junior world records! Though some of these were expected, the times turned in in the expected cases
were much better than we anticipated. All those on
'E' running two races turned in better efforts in the
second race than did those not on 'E.' This same ability to repeat when on 'E' was also noticed during
practices in the two week period before the meet.

Dr. Lambert, the noted Irish veterinarian, has
had analagous experiences with racing greyhounds
and hunting dogs. They have done very much better
after taking alpha tocopherol.[16]

An Indian report indicates that alpha tocopherol
seemed to increase the ability of soldiers at high altitudes to march and carry burdens. Obviously much
remains to be done in this general area of interest,
but it should be a fruitful field of study.

Chapter 37

VITAMIN E FOR

VETERINARY PRACTICE

There is a remarkable difference in the requirement
of vitamin E for various species of animals. For example, chicks deprived of it develop a serious disease
called encephalomalacia. Male fowls become irre-
versibly sterile. Eggs laid are much less hatchable.
Turkey perosis is tocopherol-related. Sheep and
calves develop a muscular disease, (called "stiff-lamb
disease" in the former) both types of animals developing muscular stiffness and weakness and usually dying of heart failure. Diseases in pigs (called
"yellow fat disease" and "fatal syncope") appear to be
due to the same general deficiency. Young pups of
bitches deficient in the vitamin may die of hemorrhagic complications. Yellow fat disease (steatits) in
ranch mink and kittens appears to be another example, the disease being often due to overfeeding with
rancid fish. The barn-fed cow often seems to be criti-
cally deficient in this vitamin as the calving season

nears. Fodder that has been cut when fully ripe or over-ripened or that has been stored for a long time, or cereals already ground, have lost much of their vitamin value. Hay-making itself causes significant losses of tocopherol. How much is contained in most poultry feeds is unknown. Root crops contain little of it. Alfalfa leaf meal may be able to supply all that a chicken needs—or only 5 percent of it, the meal varies so greatly in its tocopherol content.

Food elements in general use may be a factor in this type of deficiency, as in the mink disease just mentioned. For example, unsaturated fats such as cod liver oil or linseed oil are able to neutralize or destroy vitamin E in the diet and demand that more tocopherol be used concomitantly.

On the other hand bulls, bucks, rams seem to need very little alpha tocopherol, or may be better able to utilize what is already in their food.

How important this all is to the farmer may be gathered from the fact that muscular dystrophy affected about 30 percent of Michigan lambs in 1939 and a similar disease in pigs in East Prussia in 1939 caused ten times the mortality due to any other disease. The amount of milder disease of this same type may be even greater.

Heart failure of various types seems to be much commoner in domestic animals than has been suspected. It is now known to be common in cows and young calves, lambs, even in pigs and gelts. The best studies have been done on dogs and cats by Lambert of Ireland, and by many groups of American workers on lambs and cattle, but these observations have now been extended to racehorses. Lambert found that many panting, listless dogs and cats had heart disease and could be restored by giving alpha tocopherol. He has even returned incapacitated hunting dogs to the field, and has had many slow racing greyhounds become winners again on British tracks.

There is and should be wide interest in these observations amongst owners of fine pedigreed stock. Vitamin E is well known in the veterinary world but deserves even wider trial. Undoubtedly it will prove to be of major interest to owners of pedigreed stock, or pets, and to racing stables of horses or dogs. Birds fed extra amounts of tocopherols lay down a fat more resistant to rancidity and build more flavorsome meat.

Dosage must be comparable to that used in man, apparently, and as in man, must be continued indefinitely. There are many forms of cheap wheat germ oil recommended for veterinary uses. Many of these are disappointing, and are rancid or too dilute to be helpful. Rancidity at once destroys any alpha tocopherol present. Please remember this. People using this substance for their stock should use alpha tocopherol, not just any illusory oil with a deceptive label. Often the oil could scarcely contain enough alpha tocopherol to support a lazy mouse, much less a cow about to calve or a hound to hunt.

The only Canadian horse ever to win the Kentucky Derby was born, raised and raced on large doses of alpha tocopherol. Indeed, vitamin E seems to be the secret weapon of many great racehorses and human athletes.

Chapter 38

AN OUNCE OF

PREVENTION

We have always been more interested in prevention than in cure. Why should men wait to be stricken with degenerative diseases when there is now good hope of warding off many of them or of ameliorating the bad effects of such as are already well under way?

Admittedly, one cannot ward off broken legs but must take them as they come. One cannot ward off pneumonia, perhaps, or the lightning bolt. But medicine has gradually developed immunizations against many such infectious diseases as smallpox and diptheria, and lately antibiotics have come to our aid to combat infection in general as soon as it shows its ugly face. The degenerative diseases remain largely untouched—and we age, develop hardened arteries and brains, lose our hair and our sight, notice our skin wrinkle and sag as if Medicine had nothing to say about all this.

We believe that there is now hope for the cardiovascular degenerations, at least. We all know what alpha tocopherol can do for these conditions once they have developed. And the outstanding characteristic of such food factors as the vitamins is that they prevent what they relieve. In short, why wait for your coronary? Why not prevent it?

One uses vitamin B-1 to prevent neuritis because it has been found to cure neuritis.

One uses vitamin B-2 to prevent catilosis, which has such symptoms as raw tongue and lips and indicates B-2 (riboflavin) deficiency.

One uses niacin to prevent pellagra because it has been found so valuable in treating pellagra.

One uses vitamin C to prevent scurvy because it has long been known to cure scurvy.

One uses vitamin D to prevent rickets because it has long been known to cure rickets.

One uses vitamin K to prevent hemorrhagic disease of the newborn because it cures hemorrhagic disease of the newborn.

Could vitamin E (alpha tocopherol) be the sole exception to the rule that vitamins tend to prevent what they relieve?

Here is the most helpful thing to be said about the prevention of these cardiovascular degenerative diseases since they were first recognized.

We know statistically that coronary heart disease kills an increasing number each year. Does one take a bigger chance awaiting his coronary clot or taking out the insurance policy that is alpha tocopherol?

People complain: "Does everyone need to take

alpha tocopherol? Isn't this treatment too expensive? If I take it, will I ever be able to discontinue its use?"

We think that everyone needs alpha tocopherol. In some instances it is vitally important, such as for the maintenance routine of any diabetic. Alpha tocopherol costs no more than other food, and life is cheap at the price. Of course, one must take it as long as he lives, just as one would continue eating any other food item. We know no other factor more versatile nor more valuable in the body's economy.

CURRICULUM VITAE

Evan V. Shute, *Doctor of Medical Sciences*
Medical Director, Shute Institute, London,
Ontario, Canada

Diplomate of the American Board of Obstetrics and
  Gynecology
Fellow of the Royal College of Surgeons of Canada
Past President of the Canadian Society for the Study of
  Fertility
Member of the Canadian Physiological Society
Member of the American Society for the Study of Sterility
Member of the British Society of Endocrinology
Fellow of the American Geriatrics Society
Fellow of the Royal Society of Medicine
Member, and Silver Medallist of the American Association
  of Abdominal Surgeons
Winner of Tom Spies Award of International Academy
  for Preventive Medicine
Member New York Academy of Sciences
Editor, the *Summary*

THE CLINICAL

HISTORY OF VITAMIN E

1922 discovered independently by Evans and Bishop at the University of California and Sure at the University of Arkansas.

called the fertility vitamin (vitamin X) since it enabled rat pregnancies which would otherwise have miscarried to be carried to term.

1932 Vogt-Moller, a Danish veterinarian, suggested it be used to prevent "habitual abortion" in pregnant women.

1933 many workers began to study this proposal, including a group in London, Canada, of which Dr. E. V. Shute made one.

Chronicle of uses:

1937 placental detachment (E. V. Shute)
menopause (E. V. Shute)
angina pectoris (E. V. Shute and W. E. Shute)

1938 indolent ulcer (Leranth and Frank in Hungary)
allergy to vitamin E (E. V. Shute)
painful menses (E. V. Shute)
itching and degenerations of skin of female genitalia and anus (E. V. Shute)
wound healing (Bartolomucci in Italy)

1939 kidney disease (E. V. Shute)
toxemia of pregnancy (E. V. Shute)

1942 male reproductive cells (E. V. Shute)
dilatation of capillaries (E. V. Shute)
prematurity (E. V. Shute and W. B. Shute)

1943 sclerodema (Szasz in Hungary)
scarring of the cornea of the eye (Stone in U.S.A.)

1944 prophylaxis of fibroid tumors of womb (E. V. Shute)
womb (E. V. Shute)

1945 diabetes mellitus (Butturini in Italy)

1946 purpura with deficiency of blood platelets (Skelton, Waud, Skinner and E. V. Shute)
periodontal diseases of the gum and mouth (W. E. Shute, A. Vogelsang and E. V. Shute)
diabetes mellitus (W. E. Shute, A. Vogelsang and E. V. Shute)

1947 rheumatic heart disease (W. E. Shute, A. Vogelsang and E. V. Shute)
hypertensive heart disease (W. E. Shute, A. Vogelsang and E. V. Shute)
diabetes mellitus (independently W. E. Shute, A. Vogelsang and E. V. Shute)

1948 Buerger's disease (W. E. Shute, A. Vogelsang and E. V. Shute)
clots in blood vessels (F. Skelton, W. E. Shute and E. V. Shute)
apoplexy (W. E. Shute, A. Vogelsang and E. V. Shute)

early gangrene (W. E. Shute, A. Vogelsang and E. V. Shute)

claudication (C. K. Stuart, in Canada)

burns and radiation reactions (E. V. Shute)

painful breasts (I. Smith)

1949 stimulating wound healing (W. E. Shute and E. V. Shute)

Peyronie's disease and urethral stricture (Scott and Scardino in U.S.A.)

post-operative intra-abdominal adhesions (Bellanti in Italy)

haemophilia (Prosperi and Lottini in Italy)

1950 varicose veins (W. E. Shute and E. V. Shute)

congenital heart disease (W. E. Shute)

acute rheumatic fever (W. E. Shute)

osteomyelitis (W. E. Shute and E. V. Shute)

tropical ulcer (Bierzynski in West Indies)

diabetic vulvitis (E. V. Shute)

leukoplakia of vocal cords (W. E. Shute)

granuloma annulare (Cochrane in Scotland)

X-ray burns (W. E. Shute and E. V. Shute) (also Block in U.S.A.)

lupus erythematosis (Block and also Sterzi, in U.S.A. and Italy)

1951 eyes in hypertension (Seidenari, Mars and Morpurgo in Italy)

overgrown scars (keloids) (Edgerton, Hanrahan and Davis in U.S.A.)

degeneration of the choroid coat of the eye (E. V. Shute)

peptic ulcer (Garcia in Spain)

calcinosis (Freund in U.S.A.)

muscular power (Percival in Canada)

cataract in the eye (W. E. Shute)

breaking up of red blood cells (Rose and Gyorgy in U.S.A.)

one type of bladder inflammation (Van Duzen and Mustain in U.S.A.)

1952   diffuse scarring of the lower leg (E. V. Shute)
leprosy (de Mello in Brazil)
acne vulgaris scars (W. E. Shute)

1953   brittle bones in children (W. E. Shute)
sires of defective children (E. V. Shute)
strictures in the rectum (Ant in U.S.A.)
surgical disease of the joints (Schneider in Germany)

1954   chickenpox scars (E.V. Shute)

1955   degeneration of macula of eye (Raverdino in Italy)
haemophilia (Prosperi in Italy)

1956   retrobulbar neuritis (Lee in U.S.A.)

1957   "devil's pinches" (E. V. Shute)
corneal ulcer (W. E. Shute)
mental defectives (del Giudice in Argentina)

1958   nocturnal leg pain (E. V. Shute)

1959   tumours in animals (Lambert in Ireland)
anterior poliomyelitis (E. V. Shute)

1963   infant megaloblastic anaemia (Majaj et al. in Jordan)

1964   epidermalysis bullosa (Wilson in Canada)
chronic wound sinuses (E. V. Shute)

1965   anaemia of prematures (Oski and Barness in U.S.A.)
progressive spinal muscular atrophy (Nielson in U.S.A.)

1966   pulmonary embolism (E. V. Shute)

REFERENCES

1. American Heart Association Special Committee Report quoted in *Alpha Tocopherol in Cardiovascular Disease.* 1954. Toronto: Ryerson Press. p. 25.

2. Emerson, G. A. and Lewis, J. S. 1972. International Symposium on Vitamin E. Japan.

3. Horwitt, M. K. Sept. 27 and 28, 1973. International Symposium on Vitamin E. Minneapolis.

4. Horwitt, M. K. 1976. *Am. J. Clin.*, 29: 569.

5. Hickman, K. C. D. 1948. *Rec. Chem. Progress.* Fall issue.

6. Harris, P. L., Hickman, K. C. D., Jensen, J. L. and Spies, R. O. 1946. *Am. J. Health.* 36: 155.

7. Horwitt, M. K., Harvey, I. S., and Witting, L. A. 1961. *J. Am. Dietetic Assoc.* 38: 231.

8. Herting, D. C. and Drury, E. J. E. 1969. *J. Agric. Food Chem.*, 17: 785.

9. Shute, E. V. et al. *Summary.* The Shute Foundation for Medical Research. Canada: London, Ontario.

10. *Alpha Topcopherol in Cardiovascular Disease.*

11. Furman, S., Escher, D. J., Solomon, A., and Schwedel, J. B. 1966. *Ann. Surg.*, 164: 465.

12. Ochsner, A. 1968. *Postgrad. Med.* July, p. 94.

13. Butturini, V. 1950. *Gior. de Clin. Med.* 31: 1.

14. Vogt-Moller, P. L. 1932, *The Lancet.*

15. Percival, L. 1951. *Sun mary*, 3: 55.

16. Lambert, N. H. 1947 *Vet. Rec.*, 27: 355.

SUGGESTED ADDITIONAL READING

ON THE SUBJECT OF VITAMIN E

Adams, Ruth and Murray, Frank. 1971. *Vitamin E, Wonder Worker of the 70s*. New York: Larchmont Books.

Bailey, Herbert. 1968. *Your Key to a Healthy Heart*. New York: Arco Publishing Co.

Di Cyan, Erwin. 1972. *Vitamin E and Aging*. New York: Pyramid Books.

Di Cyan, Erwin. 1974. *Vitamins in Your Life*. New York: Simon & Schuster.

Murray, Frank. 1977. *Program Your Heart for Health*. New York: Larchmont Books.

Shute, Evan V. and staff. *Common Questions about Vitamin E*. Canada: Temside Press, London, Ontario.

Shute, Wilfrid E. 1975. *The Complete, Updated Vitamin E Book*. New Canaan, Ct.: Keats Publishing.

Shute, Wilfrid E. and Taub, Harald. 1969. *Vitamin E for Ailing and Healthy Hearts*. New York: Pyramid Books.

INDEX